Ethical Issues in Cancer Patient Care

Cancer Treatment and Research

Steven T. Rosen, M.D., *Series Editor*

Sugarbaker, P.H. (ed): Management of Gastric Cancer. 1991. ISBN 0-7923-1102-7.

Pinedo H.M., Verweij J., Suit, H.D., (eds): Soft Tissue Sarcomas: New Developments in the Multidisciplinary Approach to Treatment. 1991. ISBN 0-7923-1139-6.

Ozols, R.F., (ed): Molecular and Clinical Advances in Anticancer Drug Resistance. 1991. ISBN 0-7923-1212-0.

Muggia, F.M. (ed): New Drugs, Concepts and Results in Cancer Chemotherapy 1991. ISBN 0-7923-1253-8.

Dickson, R.B., Lippman, M.E. (eds): Genes, Oncogenes and Hormones: Advances in Cellular and Molecular Biology of Breast Cancer. 1992. ISBN 0-7923-1748-3.

Humphrey, G. Bennett, Schraffordt Koops, H., Molenaar, W.M., Postma, A., (eds): Osteosarcoma in Adolescents and Young Adults: New Developments and Controversies. 1993. ISBN 0-7923-1905-2.

Benz, C. C., Liu, E. T. (eds): Oncogenes and Tumor Suppressor Genes in Human Malignancies. 1993. ISBN 0-7923-1960-5.

Freireich, E.J., Kantarjian, H., (eds): Leukemia: Advances in Research and Treatment. 1993. ISBN 0-7923-1967-2.

Dana, B. W., (ed): Malignant Lymphomas, Including Hodgkin's Disease: Diagnosis, Management, and Special Problems. 1993. ISBN 0-7923-2171-5.

Nathanson, L. (ed): Current Research and Clinical Management of Melanoma. 1993. ISBN 0-7923-2152-9.

Verweij, J., Pinedo, H. M., Suit, H. D. (eds): Multidisciplinary Treatment of Soft Tissue Sarcomas. 1993. ISBN 0-7923-2183-9.

Rosen, S. T., Kuzel, T. M. (eds): Immunoconjugate Therapy of Hematologic Malignancies. 1993. ISBN 0-7923-2270-3.

Sugarbaker, P. H. (ed): Hepatobiliary Cancer. 1994. ISBN 0-7923-2501-X. .

Rothenberg, M. L. (ed): Gynecologic Oncology: Controversies and New Developments. 1994. ISBN 0-7923-2634-2.

Dickson, R. B., Lippman, M. E. (eds.): Mammary Tumorigenesis and Malignant Progression. 1994. ISBN 0-7923-2647-4.

Hansen, H. H., (ed): Lung Cancer. Advances in Basic and Clinical Research. 1994. ISBN 0-7923-2835-3.

Goldstein, L.J., Ozols, R. F. (eds.): Anticancer Drug Resistance. Advances in Molecular and Clinical Research. 1994. ISBN 0-7923-2836-1.

Hong, W.K., Weber, R.S. (eds.): Head and Neck Cancer. Basic and Clinical Aspects. 1994. ISBN 0-7923-3015-3.

Thall, P.F. (ed): Recent Advances in Clinical Trial Design and Analysis. 1995. ISBN 0-7923-3235-0.

Buckner, C. D. (ed): Technical and Biological Components of Marrow Transplantation. 1995. ISBN 0-7923-3394-2.

Winter, J.N. (ed.): Blood Stem Cell Transplantation. 1997. ISBN 0-7923-4260-7.

Muggia, F.M. (ed): Concepts, Mechanisms, and New Targets for Chemotherapy. 1995. ISBN 0-7923-3525-2.

Klastersky, J. (ed): Infectious Complications of Cancer. 1995. ISBN 0-7923-3598-8.

Kurzrock, R., Talpaz, M. (eds): Cytokines: Interleukins and Their Receptors. 1995. ISBN 0-7923-3636-4.

Sugarbaker, P. (ed): Peritoneal Carcinomatosis: Drugs and Diseases. 1995. ISBN 0-7923-3726-3.

Sugarbaker, P. (ed): Peritoneal Carcinomatosis: Principles of Management. 1995. ISBN 0-7923-3727-1.

Dickson, R.B., Lippman, M.E. (eds.): Mammary Tumor Cell Cycle, Differentiation and Metastasis. 1995. ISBN 0-7923-3905-3.

Freireich, E.J, Kantarjian, H. (eds.): Molecular Genetics and Therapy of Leukemia. 1995. ISBN 0-7923-3912-6.

Cabanillas, F., Rodriguez, M.A. (eds.): Advances in Lymphoma Research. 1996. ISBN 0-7923-3929-0.

Miller, A.B. (ed.): Advances in Cancer Screening. 1996. ISBN 0-7923-4019-1.

Hait , W.N. (ed.): Drug Resistance. 1996. ISBN 0-7923-4022-1.

Pienta, K.J. (ed.): Diagnosis and Treatment of Genitourinary Malignancies. 1996. ISBN 0-7923-4164-3.

Arnold, A.J. (ed.): Endocrine Neoplasms. 1997. ISBN 0-7923-4354-9.

Pollock, R.E. (ed.): Surgical Oncology. 1997. ISBN 0-7923-9900-5.

Verweij, J., Pinedo, H.M., Suit, H.D. (eds.): Soft Tissue Sarcomas: Present Achievements and Future Prospects. 1997. ISBN 0-7923-9913-7.

Walterhouse, D.O., Cohn, S. L. (eds.): Diagnostic and Therapeutic Advances in Pediatric Oncology. 1997. ISBN 0-7923-9978-1.

Mittal, B.B., Purdy, J.A., Ang, K.K. (eds.): Radiation Therapy. 1998. ISBN 0-7923-9981-1.

Foon, K.A., Muss, H.B. (eds.): Biological and Hormonal Therapies of Cancer. 1998. ISBN 0-7923-9997-8.

Ozols, R.F. (ed.): Gynecologic Oncology. 1998. ISBN 0-7923-8070-3.

Noskin, G. A. (ed.): Management of Infectious Complications in Cancer Patients. 1998. ISBN 0-7923-8150-5

Bennett, C. L. (ed.): Cancer Policy. 1998. ISBN 0-7923-8203-X

Benson, A. B. (ed.): Gastrointestinal Oncology. 1998. ISBN 0-7923-8205-6

Tallman, M.S. , Gordon, L.I. (eds.): Diagnostic and Therapeutic Advances in Hematologic Malignancies. 1998. ISBN 0-7923-8206-4

von Gunten, C.F. (ed.): Palliative Care and Rehabilitation of Cancer Patients. 1999. ISBN 0-7923-8525-X

Burt, R.K., M.M. Brush (eds): Advances in Allogeneic Hematopoietic Stem Cell Transplantation. 1999. ISBN 0-7923-7714-1

Angelos, P. (ed): Ethical Issues in Cancer Patient Care 2000. ISBN 0-7923-7726-5.

Ethical Issues in Cancer Patient Care

Edited by

Peter Angelos, M.D., Ph.D.

Assistant Professor of Surgery
Assistant Professor of Medical Ethics and
Humanities

Robert H. Lurie Comprehensive Cancer
Center

Northwestern University Medical School
Chicago, Illinois

1999 Kluwer Academic Publishers

Distributors for North, Central and South America:
Kluwer Academic Publishers
101 Philip Drive
Assinippi Park
Norwell, Massachusetts 02061 USA

Distributors for all other countries:
Kluwer Academic Publishers Group
Distribution Centre
Post Office Box 322
3300 AH Dordrecht, THE NETHERLANDS

Library of Congress Cataloging-in-Publication Data

99-049245
CIP

For Meghan, Christian, Audrey, and especially Grace.

CONTENTS

List of Contributors

Peter Angelos, M.D., Ph.D. Assistant Professor of Surgery; Assistant Professor of Medical Ethics and Humanities, Robert H. Lurie Comprehensive Cancer Center, Northwestern University Medical School, 300 E. Superior Street, Tarry 11-703, Chicago, IL 60611

Charles Bennett, M.D., Ph.D. Director HSR & D (Health Services Research & Development), VA Chicago Health Systems, Lakeside, Associate Professor Medicine, Robert H. Lurie Comprehensive Cancer Center of Northwestern University, 400 E. Ontario, Suite 204, Chicago, IL 60611.

James Bresnahan, S.J., J.D., L.L.M. , Ph.D. Professor, Emeritus of Medical Ethics and Humanities and of Medicine, Northwestern Unversity, Ward Bldg. 3-130, CH W 117, 303 E. Chicago Avenue, Chicago, IL 60611

Tod Chambers, Ph.D. Assistant Professor of Medical Ethics and Humanities and of Medicine, Northwestern University, Ward Bldg. 3-130 CH W 117, 303 E. Chicago Avenue, Chicago, IL 60611.

Christopher Daugherty, M.D. Assistant Professor of Medicine, Section of Hematology/Oncology, Department of Medicine, Associate Faculty Center for Clinical Medical Ethics, University of Chicago, Vice-Chair of Institutional Review Board, University of Chicago, 5841 S. Maryland, MC-2115, Chicago, IL 60637-1470.

Sarah E. Friebert, M.D. Associate Professor of Pediatrics, Pediatric Hematology/Oncologist, St. Vincent Mercy Medical/Mercy Children's Hospital, Associate Medical Director and Pediatric Director at Hospice of Western Reserve, Case Western Reserve, 300 E. 185th Street, Cleveland, OH 44119

Samuel Hellman, M.D. A.N. Pritzker Distinguished Services Professor, Department of Radiation of Cellular Oncology. University of Chicago, 5758 S. Maryland, D CAM Rm 1339, MC 9001, Chicago, IL 60637-1470.

Eric Kodish, M.D. Associate Professor of Pediatrics, Oncology, and Biomedical Ethics. Case Western Reserve, Rainbow, Babies and Children's Hospital, Room 310, 11100 Euclid Avenue, Cleveland, OH 44106.

Jeanne Martinez, R.N., M.P.H., CRNH Coordinator of Center for Palliative Medicine, Education and Research, 400 E. Ontario, Suite 204, Chicago, IL 60611

John M. Merrill, M.D. Associate Professor, Clinical/Medicine Hematology/Oncology. Robert H. Lurie Comprehensive Cancer Center, 676 N. St. Clair, Suite 2140, Chicago, IL 60611-2998

Kathryn Montgomery, Ph.D. Professor of Medical Ethics and Humanities and of Medicine, Program Director, Northwestern Unversity, Ward Bldg. 3-130, CH W 117, 303 E. Chicago Avenue, Chicago, IL 60611

Gary Shapiro, M.D. Associate Professor of Medicine, Head, Medical Oncology Division, Milwaukee, University of Wisconsin Medical School, Sinai Samaritan Medical Center, 945 N. 12th Street, P.O. Box 342, Milwaukee, WI 53201

Charles von Gunten, M.D., Ph.D. Medical Director, Center for Palliative Studies, 4311 Third Avenue, San Diego, CA 92103-1407.

Preface

This book addresses a variety of ethical issues that arise in the care of oncology patients. Many volumes have been written on medical ethics in the past 30 years. However, few have focused on ethical issues specific to the care of cancer patients. This book brings together such a focused examination.

The contributors are experienced clinicians, ethicists, medical humanists, and medical educators. The issues raised have direct relevance to the care of oncology patients in treatment as well as research settings.

The chapters address issues that are central to contemporary medical practice and medical ethics inquiry. Any practicing clinician will be well aware of the problems of communication and how uncertainty, cross-cultural issues, and religious influences can impact patient care. The limits of care and the role of advance directives and palliative care are common issues that must be addressed in treating patients at the end of life. For oncologists and oncology patients, participation in clinical trials may be a thorny topic, especially when phase I clinical trials are being considered. The impact of managed care and reimbursement issues cannot be avoided in the contemporary patient care and similarly cannot be neglected when considering the ethical ramifications raised. No discussion of ethics in oncology can be complete without attention to the specific challenges raised by the pediatric patient with cancer. All of these topics are explored by the contributors to this book.

This volume will have direct importance for practicing physicians, nurses, and other care- givers who take care of cancer patients. In addition, medical students, medical educators, and ethicists should find this book of interest as well.

A book such as this is the result of the efforts of many people. I am appreciative of the hard work of all of the contributors. I would like to thank Steven Rosen, M.D., the series editor of *Cancer Treatment and Research*, for his insights in realizing the importance of a volume on medical ethics in the series. Melissa Ramondetta and her staff at Kluwer have been helpful and patient over the previous months. Sandra Kuipers has helped in numerous ways. Special thanks are owed to Alex Langerman for his invaluable assistance in the final manuscript preparation of this book. Of course, I would never have been able to complete a project such as this without the patience and support of my family. Thank you all.

1 PHYSICIANS AND CANCER PATIENTS: COMMUNICATION AND ADVANCE DIRECTIVES

Peter Angelos, M.D., Ph.D.

INTRODUCTION

Over the previous several decades, numerous changes have occurred in the medical care of cancer patients in the United States. Medications and technologies not previously dreamed of are now commonplace as physicians treat patients with various malignancies. In the midst of these diagnostic and therapeutic advances, another significant change has occurred in how physicians talk to patients with cancer. Just a few decades ago, physicians routinely would not disclose the diagnosis of cancer with a patient. Today, such an approach would be unthinkable to most physicians and patients in the United States. In fact, the current discussions about advance directives assume that a certain minimum level of communication between doctor and patient has occurred.

In the following chapter, we will explore the changes that have occurred in what physicians disclose to patients about their disease. A historical approach will be taken to emphasize the contrast in the level of physician-patient communication that is accepted today as standard of care as compared to that which was considered the standard in the past. Truth-telling can be seen as but one component of physician-patient communication, yet this aspect of communication is particularly illustrative of the underlying physician-patient relationship.

Truth-telling is a complex issue in communication. It involves the philosophical question of, 'What is truth?' Furthermore, it involves the historical, cultural, and social influences that affect how illness is understood by physicians and patients. In the upcoming chapters, Kathryn Hunter and Tod Chambers will address broader issues of communication and cultural influences, respectively, that affect the care of cancer patients. In the current chapter, truth-telling by physicians will be taken to mean the honest transmission of what is accepted medical knowledge at a given time. In other words, truth-telling is what doctors tell their patients about the diseases from which the patients suffer. Medical knowledge must be seen as changing. In order to be truthful, physicians must acknowledge the uncertainty of medical "facts" when they are communicated to patients.[1]

The changes in communication with cancer patients that can be traced over previous decades largely reflect the changing paradigms of the physician-patient relationship. The earlier paradigm conceived of the patient as being passive, whereas this has now shifted to a paradigm in which the patient is an active participant in the decision making. In this context, the current emphasis on advance directives can be seen as an attempt to further extend patient autonomy. Living wills and durable power of attorney for healthcare documents will be considered in relation to doctor-patient communication. Recent studies of the use of advance directives will be examined in relation to the possible benefits to patients.

THE PHYSICIAN-PATIENT RELATIONSHIP AND COMMUNICATION

Paternalism

Until recently, the longstanding paradigm model of the physician-patient relationship was that of paternalism. According to this model, the doctor was cast as the knowledgeable and concerned father, who took the active role of making decisions for the patient child. The patient took on the passive role of the child who being dependent on the physician father would allow the physician to make the most beneficial choices for him. Physicians were best positioned, according to this view, to make decisions for their patients because physicians possessed superior medical knowledge. The physician could thereby make the best decisions for patients knowing what would be of medical benefit to the patient.

This view of the physician-patient relationship assumed that *patient benefit* always was identical to *medical benefit*. In other words, when determining how to best benefit a patient, a physician needed only to consider a medical point of view. There was no need to consider the patient's particular values or goals because they were irrelevant to the issue of what decision would best treat his or her disease or illness.

Truth and Communication

Because the physicians were the ones making decisions for their patients, under the paternalism paradigm, there was little need for physicians to communicate potentially upsetting information to patients, whether it be the diagnosis of cancer or any other detailed information relating to the patient's medical condition or treatment. Review of the literature of the 1950's and 1960's suggests that the majority of physicians would not discuss a diagnosis of cancer with a patient. In

1953, Fitts and Ravdin surveyed 442 Philadelphia physicians regarding what they tell patients with cancer.[2] Of the respondents, 57% said that they "usually do not tell," and 12% said they "never" tell the diagnosis of cancer to the patient. In a 1961 study from Michael Reese Hospital in Chicago, Oken reported similar results with 88% of physicians interviewed stating that they generally did not tell the patient a diagnosis of cancer.[3] The justification for not communicating such information to patients was that it might lead the patient to lose hope.

In contrast to the widespread practices of physicians in not communicating a diagnosis of cancer, a number of studies show that patients, even at that time, did not agree with the approaches taken by physicians. In each of three separate studies of cancer patients or their families published between 1950 and 1957, at least 81% of patients wanted to know of their diagnosis of cancer.[4,5,6]

The discrepancy between what physicians reported they told patients about cancer and what patients wanted to know is not an isolated finding within the United States. In 1964, 350 Christian Japanese doctors were asked what they tell patients regarding a diagnosis of cancer. Of the 132 respondents, only 16% of the physicians reported telling the patient the diagnosis, while 76% answered that they would only tell the diagnosis to the patient's family and not directly to the patient.[7] In comparison, a 1963 survey of 4300 Japanese citizens revealed that 90% wanted to be told their diagnosis if they were to develop cancer.[8]

Of course, if physicians were not even willing to disclose the diagnosis to their patients, we can assume that they certainly would not discuss any negative information regarding their care and treatment.

SIGNS OF CHANGE

In recent decades, many changes in society have occurred which have affected the paternalistic paradigm of the physician-patient relationship. For instance, people came to increasingly question authority. Physicians, seen as figures of authority, were questioned and "what the doctor said" came to be seen as just a recommendation rather than a decision. The rise of the consumer rights movement carried over to other aspects of society and patients became dissatisfied with paternalism as a paradigm for medical care.

Increasingly, patients sought to assert control over their bodies by participating in medical decision making. In competition with paternalism, respect for patient autonomy arose as a new paradigm for medical care.[9] According to this concept of the physician-patient relationship, decision making had to be shared between physician and patient. The patient's values and choices needed to be respected in determining what would be best for the patient. As such, *patient* benefit became distinct from *medical* benefit. In order to determine what would most benefit a patient, the patient's values needed consideration. For example, a physician could no longer assume that prolonging life was the best thing for every patient. Depending on the particular patient's values, a shorter life with less pain or suffering might be considered the most beneficial for a particular patient. By according respect for patient autonomy a central role in medical decision making, the paternalistic paradigm of the relationship needed to be exchanged for a shared decision making paradigm.

Shared decision making required physicians to not only tell their patients of their diagnosis, but also to give them more detailed information regarding their prognosis and treatment options. Without such information, patients could not participate in decision making with their physicians. It is impossible to determine whether this shift to shared decision making resulted in physicians communicating more information to patients or whether the drive for more information led to the shift toward shared decision making. Regardless of the temporal relationship between these changes, they occurred in close conjunction with one another.

The dramatic changes that occurred in doctor-patient communication can be seen by examining the 1979 study by Novack *et al.*[10] These investigators, also working at Michael Reese Hospital in Chicago, administered a virtually identical survey to the one reported by Oken in 1961. In contrast to Oken's finding that 88% of physicians generally did not tell the patient of a diagnosis of cancer, the later investigators found that 98% of physicians reported that their general policy was to tell the patient of a diagnosis of cancer.

This dramatic change within a single institution reflects the many influences which changed the physician-patient relationship. Moreover, given that the prevalent paradigm for the physician-patient relationship remains to be that of shared decision making, the Novack study provides evidence that in contemporary practice, there are few physicians who withhold the diagnosis of cancer from their patients. That this appears to be the preferred approach is supported by numerous authors in the medical ethics literature who have suggested that there can be little, if any, justification for withholding the diagnosis of cancer (or anything else) from a patient.[9,11,12,13]

The importance of shared decision making has so fully supplanted the previous paternalism that few physicians would ever think of not communicating a diagnosis of cancer with a patient. This trend is reflected in contemporary medical literature where there is a marked absence of articles questioning whether patients should be told of their diagnosis.[14] Rather, the current focus has been on *how much* to tell a patient. In other words, today's debated topic has become the completeness of disclosure which should be provided about prognosis and treatment options.

Once it is generally accepted that patients should be allowed to make informed decisions regarding their medical care, there is the issue of *how much* information is warranted and whether statistical data should be included in the information given to patients. Despite the general acceptance of the importance of patients making informed decisions, evidence suggests that some patients may be given less information than they would like. A 1982 national survey found that 96% of Americans wished to be told if they have cancer and 85% said that they wanted a "realistic estimate" of their life expectancy if their type of cancer "usually leads to death in less than a year.[15] Nevertheless, in the same year, when faced with a patient who had confirmed lung cancer at an advanced stage, only 13% of physicians surveyed said that they would give the patient a "straight statistical prognosis." Twenty-eight percent of physicians stated that they would merely tell patients that the prognosis was uncertain, but that "in most cases people live no longer than a year."[15] These numbers suggest that even though patients are told of their diagnosis, they may still lack the detail of information that they want to make decisions.

How much should patients be told about poor prognoses?

The issue of "how much information is enough was raised formally in a lawsuit involving a patient with recurrent pancreatic carcinoma.[16]   In his insightful examination of this case, George J. Annas describes the central issue as, "whether the law should require physicians to report statistical life-expectancy data to their patients in cases of illness that is likely to be terminal."[17]   Although some of the legal issues raised in the case are beyond our scope of interest for this chapter, the case is worthwhile to review because of the questions raised regarding what the patient was told.

The Case of Miklos Arato[18]

A 43 year old electrical contractor undergoing exploratory laparotomy was found to have a tumor in the tail of the pancreas. The surgeon resected the tumor and on pathological evaluation, it was found to be two centimeters in size with two out of twelve resected lymph nodes positive for metastases. (This finding portended a poor prognosis.) After surgery, the surgeon told Mr. Arato and his wife that he thought all the tumor had been removed and referral was made to an oncologist. (One might consider at this point whether the lack of discussion of Mr. Arato's prognosis by the surgeon is problematic.)

The patient was subsequently evaluated by an oncologist. During the initial evaluation, the Mr. Arato filled out an 18-page survey in the physician's office. He answered "yes" to the question, "If you are seriously ill now or in the future, do you want to be told the truth about it?" The patient was told that there was substantial chance of recurrence, and that a recurrence would mean that the cancer is incurable. The oncologist recommended chemotherapy and radiation treatments on an experimental protocol, even though he acknowledged to the patient that there is a substantial chance of recurrence.   The oncologist was neither asked for, nor volunteered a prognosis. (Again, the expected prognosis was not discussed with Mr. Arato or his wife.)

While participating in the clinical trial and receiving treatment, nine months after the initial diagnosis of carcinoma was made, a recurrence was detected. Even though the physicians treating Mr. Arato believed that his life expectancy could be measured in months, they did not tell him so. The patient died three months later.

After his death, the wife and two adult children brought suit against the surgeon and oncologist alleging that the patient was never told that approximately 95% of the patients with pancreatic cancer die within five years. They claimed that Mr. Arato would have made different decisions regarding his business and his choice to participate in the clinical trial if he had been given a "statistical prognosis."

The doctors justified nondisclosure of statistical prognosis largely on grounds of medical paternalism. They claimed that reporting extremely high mortality rates might, "deprive a patient of any hope of a cure."[19] The physicians noted that in over 70 visits with them over a one year period, the patient avoided ever specifically asking about his own life expectancy and this indicated that he did not want to know the information. In addition, all the physicians testified that the statistical life expectancy of a group of patients has little predictive value for a specific patient.

Upon appeal to the California Supreme Court the case was ultimately decided in favor of the physicians. However, the legal decision reached is less important than the questions raised. Specifically, what does it mean to truly inform a patient? Must this include statistical data which may or may not have predictive value for the patient? Treatments are not begun on patients without informed consent. Does a patient need to be given statistics in order to be fully informed? Certainly there is much more to good communication than the recitation of statistics. Physicians must be sensitive to the patients' values and expectations (whether they be reasonable or not).

In the *Arato* case, a good physician-patient relationship was never established and thus good communication was not achieved. Doctors never addressed Mr. Arato's assumptions regarding his life expectancy. At the same time, Mr. Arato did not uphold his side of the relationship. He should have played a more active role in seeking information about his prognosis if he were making significant business decisions based on his assumptions about his life expectancy.

Often a lawsuit is a good indication of a problem with a relationship. In the *Arato* case, the physician-patient relationship never developed to the point where good communication between the parties was possible. The most important lesson to be learned from this case is that truth-telling can only come if a good physician-patient relationship is present.

Quirt and co-authors have shown that doctors often are poor judges of the extent to which their patients actually understand their prognosis.[20] Nevertheless, the better the physician-patient relationship, the more sensitive the physicians can be to the patient's and the family's expectations, and the more likely a physicians and patient will have an effective discussion.

EXTENDING PATIENT AUTONOMY: ADVANCE DIRECTIVES

In the previous paragraphs, we have traced changes in physician-patient communication from the paternalistic approach to the one of shared decision making. Over the last two decades the emphasis on respect for patient autonomy has led to the concept of advance directives. Advance directives commonly take the form of a living will or durable power of attorney for healthcare document. These instruments may be seen as methods for patients to extend autonomy into periods of their lives when they are not competent to make choices.

Living Wills and Durable Power of Attorney for Healthcare

Just as a physician has a moral obligation to abide by a competent patient's choices, a physician also has a moral obligation to abide by the choices designated in an advance directive. If the advance directive takes the form of a living will, the patient has defined a set of circumstances and therapies that are not acceptable. For example, a patient with widely metastatic breast cancer and recurrent malignant pleural effusions may decide that should she does not want her life prolonged in the event she is in need of intubation and long term ventilation. Even if the patient is not competent at the time that intubation and ventilation are required, the choices that she made earlier in refusing such therapy can be acted respected. If the advance directive takes the form of a durable power of attorney for healthcare document, rather than setting forth guidelines for choices of therapy, the patient designates the person that will make decisions for him or her once the patient can no longer do so.

Although advance directives have only become widely discussed in the medical ethics literature over the last ten to fifteen years, they are not a new development. In fact, living wills and durable power of attorney for healthcare documents are best thought of as simply *formal* advance directives. In contrast, *informal* advance directives are the instructions that patients have been giving family members and friends for decades as guides to what the patient would want done in certain situations. For example, a 70 year old man having an abdominal aortic aneurysm repaired may have never filled out any documents or forms, but by telling family members that he would never want to be kept alive on dialysis, he has clear informal advance directives.

The Patient Self-determination Act

The benefits of formalizing one's choices so that family, friends, and physicians abide by one's choices have made formal advance directives increasingly appealing to many patients. Furthermore, the Patient Self-determination Act (PSDA) has recently encouraged more widespread use of advance directives.[21] This federal regulation of 1991 mandates that any hospital participating in Medicare ensure that all patients admitted to the hospital be asked if they have an advance directive and given information about advance directives.

Despite the PSDA and efforts to increase the use of advance directives, several studies have shown that among large groups of patients, advance directives are not widely used and have not significantly affected patient care.[22,23,24] There are several possible reasons for the lack of use and effectiveness of advance directives in these studies. First, not enough patients have seriously considered the possibility that they may need an advance directive. Thus, too few patients have an advance directive. Second, even if they have an advance directive, few patients bring them to the hospital or inform their physicians that they have one. Finally, the PSDA itself may be poorly conceived as a means of increasing advance directive use. The PSDA requires information about advance directives to be given to patients at the time they are admitted to the hospital if they do not already have an advance directive. In the midst of a hospital admission, a patient may be poorly prepared to have the types of thoughtful discussions with family, friends, or physicians that are necessary to implement an advance directive.

Advance Directives and the Cancer Patient

Although the advantages of advanced directives are obvious, they are not widely used at the present time. Their lack of use among cancer patients is rather surprising. One might expect to find greater use of advance directives among cancer patients. In contrast to the average person, most patients with cancer have at least considered the possibility of their mortality. Furthermore, they have often had numerous interactions with physicians and other health care providers. There is evidence, however, to suggest that even among patients with cancer, few use advance directives.

In their review of patients undergoing esophagogastrectomy for esophageal cancer and Whipple procedure for pancreatic cancer, Angelos and Johnston found that very few patients had an advance directive at the time of admission for surgery.[25] This finding is surprising because the assumption would be that patients with malignancies undergoing elective high-risk surgical procedures might be best situated to benefit from an advance directive.

Even when patients have thought about and have advance directives, the physicians may not always aware of them. Lamont has reported that even if oncology patients have discussed their wishes with family members and even if they have formal advance directives, they often do not share that information with their oncologists.[26]

Undoubtedly psychological factors on the part of physicians and patients often impede discussions of advance directives among patients with cancer. Physicians may not want to raise the issue for fear that patients will be upset about the discussion of end-of-life issues. Patients may not want physicians to believe that they are "giving up."

These factors, however, should not be allowed to impede the full use of advance directives. In reality, having an advance directive may empower the patient knowing that he can fully control his treatment and care until the very end. Not only do advance directives grant patients autonomy at the end of life, they can be used as a stepping off point for patients and physicians to discuss issues which may become relevant at a later stage of the disease, thereby laying the foundation for continued discussion.

Patients may benefit even more if these discussions involve both the primary physician and the oncologist.[27] By starting these discussion early, the patient then has the opportunity to discuss the issues with different physicians as well as family or friends over a longer period of time. This, then is a strong argument for consistently raising the issue of advance directives early in the care of patients with cancer.

If psychological factors make it difficult for a treating physician to raise the issues relating to advance directives, perhaps someone other than the physician who is involved in the patient's care should initially raise the topic. For example, a nurse or social worker might be able to begin the discussion with the expectation that the physician and patient will continue the dialogue. By so doing, patients and physicians might be more consistently able to have the important discussions necessary for an advance directive to be useful.

CONCLUSIONS

Over the preceding pages we have explored the changing paradigms of the physician-patient relationship and how physician-patient communication has been affected by these paradigms. The paternalistic approach with the tradition of not disclosing any negative information to cancer patients has given way to a shared decision making approach in which patients are informed so that they can participate in the decision making process and thereby bring about optimum care. In current medical practice, patient autonomy must be respected and patients must therefore be adequately informed in order to make decisions. In this setting, the issue is not *whether* to tell a patient he or she has cancer, but *how* to best inform them of their condition and prognosis. As with so much of medical care, an individualized approach to communication with a patient is the optimum. By being sensitive to the patient's particular needs, a physician will be able to honestly and effectively provide the patient with the information needed to make good decisions.

Advance directives can be seen as an extension of respect for patient autonomy and a natural goal for physician-patient communication. Even though living wills and durable power of attorney documents are not currently widely used, they may provide benefits in the cancer patient that go beyond the measurable outcomes of duration of life or resuscitation attempts. Consideration of advance directives may provide patients the impetus to discuss significant issues with family, friends, and physicians that might otherwise be avoided. Furthermore, the presence of an advance directive might give the cancer patient a comforting sense of control over decisions that would need to be made should the patient ever lack the ability to exercise autonomy. For these reasons, physicians caring for cancer patients should consider any method possible to enable such discussions to routinely be raised with their patients.

Acknowledgements: *The author is indebted to Grace Koh Angelos for her comments on earlier drafts of this chapter.*

REFERENCES

1. Norton L. Truth, science, and the oncologist. Annals New York Acad Sci 1997;809:66-71.

2. Fitts WT Jr, Ravdin IS. What Philadelphia physicians tell patients with cancer. JAMA 1953;153:901-04.

3. Oken D. What to tell cancer patients: a study of medical attitudes. JAMA 1961;175:1120-28.

4. Kelly WD, Friesen SR. Do cancer patients want to be told? Surgery 1950;27:822-26.

5. Branch CHH. Psychiatric aspects of malignant disease. CA: Bull Can Prog 1956;6;102-04.

6. Samp RJ, Curreri AR. Questionnaire survey on public cancer education obtained from cancer patients and their families. Cancer 1957;10:382-84.

7. Matsuoka J. Whether cancer patients should be informed of their disease (in Japanese). J Japanese Cancer Therapy 1970;5:114. Cited in Akabayashi A, Fetters MD, Elwyn TS. Family consent, communication, and advance directives for cancer disclosure: a Japanese case and discussion. J Med Ethics 1999;25:296-301.

8. Akabayashi, Fetters, Elwyn, p. 297.

9. Beauchamp TL, Childress JF. *Principles of biomedical ethics*, 4th ed. New York: Oxford University Press, 1994.

10. Novack DH, Plumer R, Smith RL, Ochitil H, Morrow GR, Bennett JM. Changes in physicians' attitudes toward telling the cancer patient. JAMA 1979;241:897-900.

11. Pellegrino ED, Thomasma DC. *A philosophical basis of medical practice: toward a philosophy and ethic of healing professions.* New York: Oxford University Press, 1981.

12. Veatch RM. *A theory of medical ethics.* New York: Basic Books, 1981.

13. Katz J. *The silent world of doctor and patient.* New York: The Free Press, 1984.

14. Of interest is a recent issue of the *Annals of New York Academy of Sciences*. This entire publication dealt heavily with the issue of whether to disclose the diagnosis of cancer to patients. However, most of these articles were written by foreign contributors examining practices outside of the United States. We might glean from this that the shift from the paradigm of paternalism has not been as complete outside the United States. Surbone A, Zwitter M. Communication with the cancer patient: information and truth. Annals N Y Acad Sciences 1997;809.

15. President's Commission for the Study of Ethical Problems in Medicine and Biomedical and Behavioral Research. *Making health care decisions: the ethical and legal implications of informed consent in the patient-practitioner relationship.* Vol. 2; Appendices. Washington, DC: US Government Printing Office, 1982, pp. 245-46.

16. Arato v. Avedon, 5 Cal. 4th 1172,23 Cal. Rptr.2d 131, 858 P.2d 598 (1993).

17. Annas GJ. Informed consent, cancer, and truth in prognosis. NEJM 1994;330:223-25.

18. In the upcoming case discussion, I have borrowed from the summary of the case by Annas cited above.

19. Annas, p. 223.

20. Quirt CF, Mackillop WJ, Ginsburg AD, et al. Do doctors know when their patients don't? A survey of doctor-patient communication in lung cancer. Lung Cancer 1997;18:1-20.

21. Cox DM, Sachs GA. Advance directives and the patient self-determination act. Clin Geriatr Med 1994;10:431-43.

22. Emanuel EJ, Weinberg DS, Gonin R, et al., How well is the patient self-determination act working? An early assessment. JAMA 1993;95:619-28.

23. Teno JM, Lynn J, Phillips RS, et al., Do formal advance directives affect resuscitation decisions and the use of resources for seriously ill patients? J Clin Ethics 1994;5:23-30.

24. Silverman HJ, Tuma P, Schaeffer MH, Singh B. Implementation of the patient self-determination act in a hospital setting: an initial evaluation. Arch Internal Med 1995;155:502-10.

25. Angelos P, Johnston C. Advance directive use among patients undergoing selected high-risk surgical procedures. Qual Management Health Care 1999;7:1-3.

26. Elizabeth Lamont, "With whom will oncology patients discuss advanced care planning?" presented at The Tenth Annual Mrs. John MacLean Conference, October 30 – November 1, 1998, Chicago, Illinois.

27. Doukas DJ, Doukas MA. Considering advance directives for oncology patients. Prim Care Clin in Office Practice 1998;25:423-31.

2 INFORMATION IS NOT ENOUGH: THE PLACE OF STATISTICS IN THE DOCTOR-PATIENT RELATIONSHIP

Kathryn Montgomery, Ph.D.

INTRODUCTION

The hero of Leo Tolstoy's *The Death of Ivan Ilych* is a man of "incorruptible honesty," who prides himself on his work as an examining magistrate:

> Ivan Ilych never abused his power; he tried on the contrary to soften its expression, but the consciousness of it and of the possibility of softening its effect supplied the chief interest and attraction of his office. In his work itself...he very soon acquired a method of eliminating all considerations irrelevant to the legal aspect of the case, and reducing even the most complicated case to a form in which it would be presented on paper only in its externals, completely excluding his personal opinion of the matter, while above all observing every prescribed formality.[1]

This professional detachment was the bureaucratic ideal after the Russian judicial reform of 1861 and was no doubt an improvement on the favoritism and bribery that had preceded it. Ivan Ilych polishes it to an art, devotes his career to its perfection:

> In all this the thing was to exclude everything fresh and vital, which always disturbs the regular course of official business, and to admit only official relations with people, and then only on official grounds.... Ivan Ilych possessed this capacity to separate his real life from the official side of affairs and not mix the two in

the highest degree and by long practice and natural aptitude had brought it to such a pitch that sometimes, in the manner of a virtuoso, he would even allow himself to let the human and official relations mingle. He let himself do this just because he felt that he could at any time he chose resume the strictly official attitude again and drop the human relation. And he did it all easily, pleasantly, correctly, and even artistically.[2]

Then, with a persistent pain in his side, Ivan Ilych seeks advice from a physician and encounters a professional very like himself:

There was the usual waiting and the important air assumed by the doctor, with which he was so familiar (resembling that which he himself assumed in court), and the sounding and listening, and the questions which called for answers that were foregone conclusions and were evidently unnecessary....

The doctor...said that so-and-so indicated that there was so-and-so inside the patient, but if the investigation of so-and-so did not confirm this, then he must assume this and that. If he assumed that and that, then...and so on. To Ivan Ilych only one question was important: was his case serious or not? But the doctor ignored that inappropriate question. From his point of view it was not the one under consideration, the real question was to decide between a floating kidney, chronic catarrh, or appendicitis. It was not a question of Ivan Ilych's life or death, but one between a floating kidney and appendicitis. And that question the doctor solved brilliantly....[3]

Not entirely daunted, Ivan Ilych presses the matter:

He...rose, placed the doctor's fee on the table, and remarked with a sigh: "We sick people probably often put inappropriate questions. But tell me, in general, is this complaint dangerous, or not?"

The doctor looked at him sternly over his spectacles with one eye, as if to say: "Prisoner, if you will not keep to the questions put to you, I shall be obliged to have you removed from the court."

"I have already told you what I consider necessary and proper. The analysis may show something more." And the doctor bowed.[4]

A century and a quarter later medical care differs in many crucial ways, but every patient's most important question is still much like Ivan Ilych's: "Is this illness serious or not?" It is a question of life or death. If such questions are no longer deflected as they were by Ivan Ilych's physician, there is still wide variation in how they are answered. The patient's disease, let's say, has a five-year disease-free survival rate of 75%. Chemotherapy can increase that to 82%. These are the facts as best they are known. Good odds, as such things go. What should the physician say to the patient? How much information does the patient need? What part should statistics play in the answer that is given?

WHAT PATIENTS WANT TO KNOW

Physicians know that patients want to know a good bit about their diagnosis, but research shows they underestimate how much. Peter Angelos's study of the quality and quantity of information provided to patients with breast, colon, and pancreatic cancer suggests that two in thirteen receive too little information and that in general patients think physicians should supply more detail than physicians themselves are comfortable offering.[5] Not only do patients want more information than physicians think they do, their concepts of "enough" differ substantially. D.D. Kerrigan and colleagues found that patients awaiting elective hernia repair experienced no increase in presurgical anxiety following a very detailed account of what might go wrong during the procedure and argue that full disclosure would reduce the potential for malpractice charges without adverse consequences for the patient.[6]

The mismatch of expectation has many sources. Physicians who are confident of the therapy they can offer may be reluctant to disturb the patient, delay treatment, diminish the patient's trust and thus perhaps lessen any placebo effect that will speed recovery. These days there is increased pressure to save time and to streamline patient encounters; when physicians do attempt to inform patients more fully, there is no guarantee that information given today will be recalled tomorrow. It is not uncommon for a physician to explain a diagnosis, outline the prognosis, and describe the treatment choices only to have the patient appear never to have been given the information. When cancer is the diagnosis, there is the added burden-- one that never entirely disappears--of delivering truly bad news. Although only a handful of patients--far fewer than in the past--want *not* to know, no one really wants to hear she has cancer. Even if the cure rate were 100%, the treatment is still severe and life-altering, and the social meaning of the disease is complicated and dire. It cannot be easy to be the agent of patients' painful discovery of a shortened life, an altered body, or limited potential. Thus, it is not surprising that even for the most experienced clinicians there is often a genuine recoil from this repetitive duty to inform, especially since it is a duty that, despite its value in the patient-physician relationship, seems to have been imposed from outside the profession.[7] Physicians understandably move to spare their patients--and spare themselves in the bargain. Even a subtle reluctance is likely to affect the amount and character of the information transmitted.

INFORMATION AND REASSURANCE

The failure to provide enough information may also be fueled by the physician's sense that patients and their families are asking for more than information, perhaps something that medicine cannot provide. Sick people facing prolonged therapy need reassurance, especially when the treatment is painful, life-threatening, or toxic in itself. Most reassuring would be a sense of certainty: in particular that the treatment will work, that the patient will be cured and restored to normal life. A great many patients and their families look for this reassurance, as our culture has taught us to do, in science. Gathering information about disease and treatment choices is one way of attempting to keep hold of a sense of predictability in the world. If life eludes control, at least we can understand how it's gone awry and how best to restore normality. And, in fact, detailed biomedical information is often useful. When treatment options are evenly weighted or when a permanent loss will be the consequence of disease or treatment, it seems that every scrap of data helps in making decisions. Such information makes sense of tests, justifies adjuvant chemotherapy, and restores a sense of choice that can ease the disaster of having cancer. It may even offer hope, sustaining patients through bad times. No wonder many patients want the most minute detail.

Nevertheless, scientific information is only part of what is needed. Data must be interpreted, evidence pieced together, and information sorted for its relevance to one particular patient. Just as most physicians have found a wide middle ground between lying and "truth-dumping,"[8] so it seems possible to find a way between the stonewalling "trust me" (with a pamphlet at best) and launching into a short course in pathophysiology with a brief excursus into cell and molecular biology. The middle ground seems large enough for every physician to find a comfortable position. What is less clear is the part that statistical results of clinical studies should play in the answer that is offered to patients.

INFORMATION AND STATISTICS

The limits to biomedical information, helpful though the facts may be both for decision-making and for a sense of control, are nowhere more pointed and painful than in the use and almost unavoidable abuse of statistics. Patients in their need for certainty ask for scientific answers. What they get--or find on the Internet--is probabilities. Chance. The numbers are, after all, "the facts"--or their most nearly accurate representation. Yet statistics are profoundly unsatisfying. In part this is because they are perceived so subjectively. Twenty years ago Daniel Kahneman and Amos Tversky studied the psychology of risk assessment and the wide range of attitudes to risk that influence behavior. They described how the way a statement of probablity is framed influences its effect and how common decision strategies, themselves based on probabilites, lead people to do such things as overestimate the importance of very low and very high percentages.[9] Education and experience do not alter this subjectivity. In the early 1980s I kept a folder of articles and stories labeled "Sick Docs," and my favorite was by a physician at Johns Hopkins, who after he finished treatment for cancer became obsessed with the insidious threat of recurrence. His numbers were good; the chance of disease-free survival for his diagnosis was solidly in the nineties. He understood the statistics as well as anyone, but the numbers were no help. After weeks of debilitating anxiety, he realized that to rid himself of his dread and go on with his life he had to come to terms with his proud record of ranking in the very top percentiles his whole life.

Should he not have been told? Should he have been discouraged from investigating it on his own? It's hard to such restraint would have been successful, even before the Internet. Five-year disease-free survival rates are part of the lore that has been absorbed as biomedicine has become the folk medicine of the West. Even twenty years ago, survival statistics, the facts about recurrence, had entered the consciousness of the average citizen without a medical degree. These days patients ask physicians whether they will recover from their disease, knowing that clinical studies offer the best available data. They expect to hear the numbers that pertain to them and their diagnosis. It's science after all. The beauty of statistics is that they provide a scientific answer; they represent a sometimes difficult but desirable honesty. They sum up the most, the best that's known about a disease and its stages. They are the best science can do. Surely they should answer the patient's most pressing question.

But despite their honesty, numbers deceive. Statistics, however helpful, are inevitably limited and misleading. "Does it look bad for me?" Statistics don't say. Survivors survive entirely; those who die are completely dead. No one survives 82%--with the grossly literal exception of amputees. Nor does the number predict disease-free time. Although it can happen, a person with a 82% chance of surviving five years without a recurrence is unlikely to find the disease recurring a month and a half into the fifth year, when only 18% of that five years remains. No matter how promising the numbers, there is no certainty that this particular patient will do well. Except in well advanced cases when an unflinching yes is called for, there is no answer that can come close to certainty. There is no negative, no qualified answer that is certain. Not only do statistics fail to answer the life or death question patients and their families ask, they make the uncertainty painfully real. Is this the best medicine can do?

Statistics and the scientific certainty they approximate, however, are not all that patients need. Sidney Bogardus and colleagues recommend using a variety of formats--qualitative, quantitative, graphic--to communicate information about risk: numbers, words, charts.[10] Numbers alone, they argue, are not adequate. Neither is an understanding of one's assigned chance, no matter how balanced and thorough. Their strategy provides a useful remedy for the misperceptions apparently built into the psychology of numbers. But it still not likely to answer the patient's burning life or death question.

What then should a physician tell a patient? The odd thing is that while most patients want more information than they presently receive--including statistics--the facts are only a stand-in for the reassurance patients need. Statistical information not only does not necessarily provide this reassurance, it is often counter-productive. A colleague who is an oncologist says he uses statistics all the time in making clinical decisions but seldom mentions them to his patients. When, as often happens, they arrive in his office armed with printouts hot off the National Cancer Institute Web site, he suggests they not put too much stock in them: "You don't want to be like the man with his head in the oven and his feet in the refrigerator," he tells them. "His head was hot, his feet were cold, but on average he was just fine." Not that the information is especially wrong, but it is not especially useful. There is no certainty.   If he is to provide support and honest reassurance, he must use something more than statistics.

This yawning chasm between the probable facts and the need for certainty is not unique to cancer care.   Given that there is little certainty in other aspects of life-- even aspects equally governed by the laws of science (think of flying, cooking, meteorology)--why should it exist in medicine?   Reassurance, however, addresses concerns that lie behind the patient's quest for certainty.   Indeed, physicians can offer reassurance even in the most inauspicious circumstances: that their patients will be well taken care of, that they will make the best possible decisions in their case, that they will not lie to them.   Farther along, there can be reassurances about the relief of pain and about not deserting them.   Such assurances are not the manifestation of biomedical facts but of medical attention, clinical judgment, and a physician's wisdom and fidelity.   These things, too, provide human beings with a sense of control in their lives.

There are barriers to providing such non-statistical reassurance.   In the United States, the fragmented health care (non-)system and the division of clinical labor by subspecialties constitute two of them.   A third barrier, however, is more personal and well within the individual physician's power to remove.   It is the failure to acknowledge the patient's question and the temptation to avoid it altogether. Knowing that the science of medicine cannot provide anything like the certainty the patient so desperately seeks, some physicians may become cynical about such a desire, ignore it, and thereby miss an opportunity to offer a different but ultimately more valuable sort of reassurance.

How best to live one's life is the central moral question for every human being, well or ill.   A life-defining illness only sharpens the need for an answer.   Providing such answers may not be the duty of the oncologist or surgeon; but if physicians are not to be mere technicians, it is necessary at least to recognize the existence of the question.   This and some advice about ways to address the day-to-day aspects of life-threatening illness are part of a physician's work.   Such advice may be as simple as pointing out that medicine cannot do the whole work of recovery alone: even when it cures the disease, the patient will have to work hard at recovering from the illness and, with cancer, from its treatment.   Unless physicians are to become mere biotechnicians, it is never true that they have "nothing more to offer."   There are referrals, Hospice, simple presence.   Chronic and degenerative diseases impose an even clearer duty.   Dewitt Stettin, Jr.'s plea to alter subspecialty practice is as useful as the day he wrote it.   After his macular degeneration was diagnosed, the best physicians in the country, many of them his former colleagues, said they "could do nothing more for him."   His *New England Journal of Medicine* article is a damning enumeration of all the conveniences--a clever talking watch, the Kurzweil reader, Talking Books--that he was left to discover on his own.[11]

A reluctance to offer nonstatistical advice and reassurance is one of the side-effects of medicine's claim to be a science. The word "science" is noble and the aspirations it evokes are praiseworthy, but the claim--and its eager acceptance by patients and society as a whole--has led to the expectation that physicians' knowledge is invariant, objective, replicable, and predictable.[12] Yet medicine is not a science, however scientific its knowledge or technological its therapies. It is, as it has always been, the diagnosis and treatment of sick people. Although biology is now the frame for much of medicine, clinical knowing is focused on the interpretation of what is happening over a course of time with a particular patient. Such knowledge is still called an opinion; the skill used in arriving at that opinion is called judgment. No one understands this better than surgeons. In their case-based, interpretive use of knowledge, physicians resemble lawyers and judges, and medical rationality resembles jurisprudence. Both are engaged in practical reasoning, which, as Aristotle observes, they also share with practitioners of navigation and moral reasoning.[13] In these practical realms of knowing, learning is particular, experiential, conventionally agreed upon, finely interpreted. Although the areas of agreement may be large, even international and transcultural, physicians (like lawyers, moral reasoners, and navigators) rely on skill and judgment that are taught and practiced, improved and clarified case by case. Without a doubt, biology grounds clinical knowledge and promotes valuable technological advance, but this simply means that medicine has both a body of essential biological knowledge and, like other practices, a fund of established practical wisdom. This double resource renders the work of clinicians far more like that of naturalists or economists or archeologists than that of biochemists or physicists.

It is this double store of knowledge and experience that patients call upon: not only the scientific facts but clinical judgment, including hunches and intuition. It is wisdom of a real-life, practical kind. Some patients may want scientific information; many more will want statistics; but all hunger for information about the world of illness they have entered. "Is it serious, doc?" What we all need to know, in one way or another, is whether we can live with our diseases. Biomedical science, millennial technology, and recent clinical attention to the care of the dying make this possible for many diagnoses to an extent (and for a length of time) unimaginable a short while ago. But to provide the reassurance patients need, physicians must be willing to go beyond the statistics.

CONCLUSION

Good physicians have always sensed what patients need. If they cannot assure them of a cure for their disease, then they can speak about the manageability of the disease or, when death is in prospect, offer reassurance about the relief of pain and their commitment not to abandon the patient. If these last are not tasks that a given specialty usually assumes, then a promise to help the patient find a physician who can make these commitments ranks a close second. Such assistance may threaten a physician's long-standing wariness about making an empathic connection with patients, but to avoid offering this help risks the opposite danger: protective detachment can harden into an unfeeling carapace that will impoverish a physician's daily experience. The work of William Branch and Anthony Suchman suggests that for many physicians connection in the patient-physician relationship is finally much less exhausting and painful than its avoidance.[14]

If contemporary practice provides no time for physician to go beyond the bare statistical information, contemporary practice must be changed. The alternative, now that the economics of medicine are laid bare, is the loss of medicine's identity as a profession rather than a business enterprise. In the short run--and at the very least--physicians who care for cancer patients need to recognize Ivan Ilych's burning question in whatever shape their patients ask it. Their best answer is not statistics, which are of little use in deciding how to live a life altered by disease and its treatment or shortened altogether. The best answer is an acknowledgment that the question is terrifyingly important. "Is my case serious or not?" "Am I going to die?" The answer is not 82%--nor even 82% certain. The answer, details of which the patient must ultimately supply, is how to live.

Acknowledgements: The author is indebted to Peter Angelos, Joel Frader, John Merrill, Henry Ruder, and especially to Beth Fine Kaplan—good clinicians all.

REFERENCES AND NOTES

1. Leo Tolstoy, "The Death of Ivan Ilych," [1886] translated by Aylmer Maude in *The Death of Ivan Ilych and Other Stories*. New York: Signet, p. 107.

2. Tolstoy, pp. 117-188.

3. Tolstoy, p. 121.

4. Tolstoy, p. 122.

5. Peter Angelos, "Patterns of Physician-Patient Communication: Results of Preliminary Studies," presented to a symposium in honor of David L. Nahrwold, Northwestern University Medical School, 27 February 1998.

6. Kerrigan DD, Thevasagayam RS, Woods TO, et al.. Who's afraid of informed consent? Brit Med J 1993;306:298-300.

7. Howard Brody, however, has made it the core of the conversational ethics he describes as essential to primary care and highly useful in sub-specialty medicine; see *The Healer's Power* (New Haven: Yale University Press, 1992).

8. The phrase has been in use for more than a decade, but there is no better illustration of it than Reynolds Price's account of being told his diagnosis, tout court, in a busy hallway of the Duke University Hospital by two young specialists who then turned and rushed off to other, more important duties: *A Whole New Life: An Illness and A Healing* (New York: Penguin/Plume, 1994).

9. Kahneman D, Tversky A. The framing of decisions and the psychology of choice. Science 1981;211:453-58. See also their earlier Judgment under uncertainty. Science 1974;185: 1124-31.

10. Bogardus ST, Holmboe E, Jekel JF. Perils, pitfalls, and possibilities in talking about medical risk. JAMA 1999;281:1037-41.

11. Stettin D. Coping with blindness. NEJM 1981; 305: 458-60.

12. Philosophers and sociologists of science have long described science as more contextual and socially constructed, but when it comes to medicine, physicians and the general public still subscribe to the now out-dated Newtonian, positivist view.

13. Aristotle, *Nicomachean Ethics* II 2, 1104a7

14. Branch WT, Suchman A. Meaningful experiences in medicine. Amer J Med 1990;88: 56-59.

3 CROSS-CULTURAL ISSUES IN CARING FOR PATIENTS WITH CANCER

Tod Chambers, Ph.D.

INTRODUCTION

In 1994, the parents of a fifteen-year-old were ordered by a California court to have their daughter undergo chemotherapy treatment for ovarian cancer. The director of the County Social Services Department stated that they asked for the court order "because clearly there was a medical neglect issue. If there is a medicine that will cure a child, and the parents do not want to use that medical treatment or medicine, then its viewed a medical neglect case."[1]

Ironically, the parents might have agreed with the director's assertion. They were Hmong refugees from Laos. They believed that they were using medicine that would cure their child of her illness; they disagreed, however, with the California officials about what her illness was and what medical treatment she needed. Many Hmong believe that certain illnesses are caused biologically, so these illnesses can be treated with Western allopathic treatments. They also hold that some illness are caused by supernatural agents, and these illnesses require the attention not of an oncologist but of a shaman. In this case, the family disagreed with the allopathic physicians' diagnosis of cancer, and they wished their daughter to be treated with traditional Hmong medicine. After her first chemotherapy session, the girl "ran away" from home. The California police believed that the family were hiding their daughter; they "admit there's little they can do if the parents don't want her found."[1] The family said that a shaman has told them that their daughter is doing well.

Cross-cultural issues can profoundly affect many of the traditional concerns of medical ethics, and, when attempting to resolve issues rooted in cultural conflicts, the moral principles developed in the United States over the past few decades do not always provide satisfactory guidance. Customarily cultural issues are perceived as something that needs to be "overcome" in order to inform patients and get their consent for procedures.[2,3] The Hmong, thus, are thought to have cultural beliefs that prevent them from fully understanding the medical issues involved in the care of this girl; in short, they have "beliefs" and we have "scientific evidence." Framing the problem in this way portrays "culture" as a foreign intrusion brought into the clinical setting. We should, however, conceive of cultural conflicts as the result of an incongruity *between* cultures.

Cultural values are often presented as a stagnant set of rules and customs. This impression leads to several problems. First, some clinicians believe that "knowing" a culture involves familiarizing oneself with a list of beliefs; cultural competence seems to entail simply knowing what "Italians believe" or what "Buddhists think." The anthropologist Margaret Lock suggests that this tendency toward seeing culture as a list of "things" is "in order to systematize and 'tidy up' culture in the same way as . . . other epidemiologic variables, such as smoking, age, gender, or fertility rates."[4] Second, culture is thought of as a straightforward entity that one is either inside or outside. In fact, people often have overlapping membership in several communities. Cultural identity for many only becomes an "issue" when they come into contact with someone who does not share their assumptions about values or worldview. Consider someone who might identity themselves as gay or Hispanic or Catholic depending with whom they are speaking. These two assumptions can mislead some clinicians to view culture as a predictor of individual behavior and as an entity lacking diversity--both unsound assumptions. An intimate familiarization with a culture often leads one to see not only the common patterns of practice among individuals but also the diversity permitted within the group.

An intimate familiarity with cultural beliefs should permit opening a conversation between patients and health care professionals. Let us say that a physician is faced with the need for surgical procedure with a new patient, who the physician knows is a devout Jehovah's Witness.[5] This knowledge of the patient's religious background (even with the information of ardent participation) should not lead the physician to assume that the patient would be unwilling to accept any form of blood products. Knowledge of the beliefs of Jehovah's Witnesses concerning blood transfusions will permit the surgeon to understand if the patient expresses distress concerning this issue, especially if the patient wishes to receive blood products if necessary. One pragmatic way to conceive of culture is as a communal pattern of life negotiated by individuals. This interaction between shared patterns and individual negotiation constitutes one of the central dynamics of our social existence. An awareness of the argument against blood transfusions, the history of these beliefs, and the diversity within the Jehovah's Witnesses community are central factors in permitting one to have a sophisticated conversation with this particular patient. Such cultural information should open a discussion with one's patient concerning how he or she has negotiated the tradition's beliefs, even if this has resulted in the patient's complete acceptance of the tradition's stances. The cultural anthropologist Clifford Geertz observes that "culture is not a power, something to which social events, behaviors, institutions, or processes can be causally attributed; it is a context, something within which they can be intelligibly .

. . described."[6] In the end, knowledge of a culture does not grant <u>predictability</u> of individual behavior but rather *understandability* of that behavior.

SOURCES OF CROSS-CULTURAL CONFLICT

One of the sources of conflict is a consequence of clinicians not having the time to learn the particular cultural beliefs of their patients. We should perhaps distinguish those conflicts that arise in caring for a single person of a different culture from those that arise in caring for a particular ethnic group in one's community. The grounds for conflict in each instance may be identical, but one cannot expect clinicians to become familiar with all the cultural beliefs that may potentially conflict with their own. However, ongoing conflicts with members of a local and numerically significant community should become a clinician's business. Two of the central themes of this chapter are that clinicians have an ongoing responsibility for being conscious of their own cultural assumptions and that they need to establish an ongoing relationship with those communities that do not share these assumptions. The issue of time remains an important one in dealing with cultural issues, but in cross-cultural issues our final concern should be toward prevention and, thus, in the end, time spent on familiarizing oneself with the cultural beliefs of one's patients can save time. In preventing conflicts, we must attend to the common sources for conflict: language, worldview, values, and ethos.

Language

The most identifiable occasion for conflict is when patients and health care professionals do not share the same language. Sometimes to communicate with their patients, clinicians must rely on a third-party. The question of who this third-party should be raises additional ethical questions and may bring forth moral problems that would not normally have arisen if the physician and patient shared the same language. Translation is usually from one of three sources 1) professionals, 2) amateurs (outsiders with no relation to the patient), or 3) intimates (family members or friends). Of the three, intimates of the patients can be the most perilous, both in making a medical diagnosis and in inadvertently raising moral issues. In some instances patients may feel certain types of information--such as sexual history and family secrets--can be told to a clinician but should not be revealed to these intimates. In recounting his medical history, a man may be willing to share with the physician information about a sexually-transmitted disease but unwilling if his wife, daughter, or neighbor is also present. Furthermore intimates can often in the act of translation add or subtract information. As many clinicians know, especially during times of emergency, intimates may be the only ones who can provide assistance in gaining a patient's consent for necessary medical interventions. Nonetheless one should not settle for intimates, for it can result in more problems than the time saved in its apparent convenience.

Even when patients and physicians share the same language, in some instances conflict in communication can still arise because they do not share the same non-verbal language. Various ethnic groups in the United States use English as their primary language yet still have difficulty communicating with one another as the result of differences in the physical space required between individuals for a trusting conversation.[7] The human body functions as a central medium for communication; One social scientist divides the different ways information is presented through the body into ten codes: bodily contact, proximity, orientation, appearance, head nods, facial expression, gestures, posture, eye contact, and non-verbal aspects of speech.[8] Body posture and gestures are also signs that are often unintended sources for conflict. The simple physical gesture of touching someone on the shoulder can, according to different cultural semiotics, be read as either "commiseration" *or* "invasion." The problem with the non-verbal aspects of communication is that often they feel "natural" to each party and not acts of communication. When these unspoken rules of communication are broken, we tend to experience them in a visceral manner; while a touch on the shoulder can be experienced as comforting and thus desired, a touch on the neck can feel offensive. Clinicians need to be aware as well that silence in some cultures does not represent a pause in communication but can itself be a meaningful form of communication.[9] We need to be aware that there is nothing "natural" about our reactions and that we have as much internalized our non-verbal language as we have the conjugation of the past perfect conditional of our native tongue.

Worldview

A "worldview" is a community's conception of the way the reality "truly is." The conflict between the Hmong and the California Social Services department occurred partly because they do not share the same worldview. In the Hmong worldview, illnesses can have both natural and supernatural causes; in the social services workers' worldview, illnesses can only be the result of a natural cause. All people have a worldview; our worldview often seems the only "reasonable" way to operate in the world, so it is difficult for a person who holds a naturalistic worldview even to accept the Hmong perspective as rational. The problem is our worldview is not a rationally constructed entity but is rationally derived from our assumptions about the way the world ultimately is. Consequently if we believe in supernatural entities--in the same way many of us were raised to believe in "germs" and "viruses"--then illness from supernatural forces may be viewed as a "natural" consequence of the way the world is.

Ethos

The ethos of a community concerns the "tone, character, and quality of their life, its moral and aesthetic style and mood."[10] An ethos, the character of our daily lives, can often be the source of conflict in health care in that often medical care in various cultures is not only built upon a view of how illness is caused but also upon the kind of lives we should be living. For example, we in the United States believe that privacy between patient and physician are essential elements of the therapeutic alliance, but such concerns as privacy are a particular expression of the Anglo ethos, which can only be understood when placed alongside other beliefs such as the importance of the individual self. The Hmong possess a different ethos of the person, one which challenges the Western notion of the radically individualized self and upon reflection may make some Anglos feel their ethos may overemphasize the individual.[11]

Values

The most common explanation for conflicts within the clinical setting is that patients possess values that are different from those of the health care professionals. In 1990, health care professionals wished to discontinue a ventilator for Helgie Wanglie, an elderly woman in a persistent vegetative state.[12] The family did not disagree with the clinicians concerning the medical facts concerning her condition; they did, however, value her life in this condition. The disagreement here did not seem to be the result of differences in language, worldview, or ethos but it appears to have been the result of a conflict over valuing the life of person in a persistent vegetative state. Although there was a hope in the discourse of bioethics that such concepts as quality of life and best interest could be determined without a need to appeal to specific cultural frameworks of values, this has proven to be an elusive goal. Does the life of patient who can experience simple pleasure but is unable to be employed or live independently represent a good quality of life? The answer to this depends largely on whether one's conception of a person is forged within the protestant ethic of work and independence. Is suffering always detrimental or is it sometimes a source for personal growth or spiritual redemption? There is no culturally neutral ranking of values. The major sources of cross-cultural conflict described in the previous section are outlined in Table 1.

Table 1: Sources for Cross-Cultural Conflict

Language
Worldview
Ethos
Values

TECHNIQUES FOR RESOLUTION

When one finds oneself caught within a conflict resulting from a cultural clash, there are some simple techniques that can guide one toward a resolution.

Active Self-Reflection

Ironically perhaps the most profitable technique for understanding another culture is first to understand one's own.

One of the reasons that cultural issues arise in the practice of medicine is that both groups in the conflict see their beliefs as self-evident and natural. W.E.B. Du Bois referred to the heightened self-consciousness of many minority ethnic groups as "double consciousness," an awareness of oneself that is entangled within the perspective of another ethnic group. Lacking this double consciousness, many Anglos feel as if they do not "have" an ethnic identity. If asked about their identity, some respond that they do not feel as if their beliefs and practices are particularly "cultural" or "ethnic." Anglo culture infuses our media, health care, jurisprudence, and educational system. The argument that we should take temporary custody of the Hmong child until she is old enough to make her decisions for herself indicates an implicit belief that allopathic medicine should be the default healing practice. Our courts tend to accept the allopathic physician's perspective as normative. We must recognize that the reason that we are not predisposed to recognize Anglos as an "ethnic" group is because the values of this group are so much a part of what is traditionally identified as "American"; consequently the addition of "Anglo" to American (as in African-American or Asian-American) can seem redundant. We need to recognize some of the patterns of the Anglo ethos and worldview; in other words, to view the culture of this dominant group as if we were observers from another culture (something that most of the members of the minority cultures in the United States already do). For the sake of space, the following observations will be limited to how Anglo culture affects the practice of medicine. A good – and often interesting – source for general observations about these cultural patterns are guides written for people who are coming to the United States to work.[13,14]

The worldview of Western allopathic medicine can generally be characterized as positivistic. Knowledge about the world is thought to be best derived through the "scientific method"; although such scholars as Kathryn Montgomery Hunter have persuasively demonstrated that medicine is not a "science,"[15,16] the desire to be thought of in this way signifies the power this perspective holds in the American worldview. Accordingly Western medicine values quantification and tends to believe the most accurate and realistic form of representation is that which can be communicated through percentages of occurrence or risk. Western medicine emphasizes the material and physical over the spiritual and the emotional. This emphasis is mirrored in how the culture values the various medical fields. The psychiatrist and cultural anthropologist Arthur Kleinman observes that there is a "cultural logic" deeply embedded in Western medicine between soft and hard fields: "Talk and cognitive activities more generally are 'soft'; procedures that enter the body . . . are 'hard.'"[17] In the United States we tend to demonstrate something's value through money, so the "hard" medical specialties (such as surgery) are highly rewarded and the "soft" specialties (such as psychiatry) are given the lowest salaries. The value placed on those items that can be clearly measured and tested is greater than items that are more ambiguous. Related to this prizing of the "hard,"

Western medicine does not admit supernatural agents as the potential cause of illness; all causes (and consequently all treatments) must be attributed to the natural world. Dwight Conquergood in his description of the Hmong worldview observes the clash of epistemologies that can result when comparing health practices across cultures:

> Many of my Hmong consultants know about my detached retina that resulted in blindness in one eye. With great fascination, they questioned me in detail about the two three-hour surgeries I underwent. I could see the incredulity in their eyes when they learned that I had subjected myself to such a bizarre (in their view) ritual. (Traditional Hmong have an aversion to surgery or any cutting on the body because they believe that tampering with the body will have negative consequences for the next reincarnation). They were not at all surprised that the surgeries did not restore my sight. But they were truly shocked that I would allow myself to be subjected to such a patently unnatural procedure not once, but twice. Like well-integrated members of most cultures, however, I have little difficulty accepting modern medicine's failure to restore my eyesight even while maintaining my belief in most of its basic assumptions. [18]

Although allopathic medicine may seem to be a monologic practice, its application is contingent upon specific cultural beliefs. Lynne Payer, a journalist, suggests that even in societies that share the allopathic tradition of healing, cultural assumptions arise in surprising ways. She observes, for example, that there seems a link between the French treatments for cancer (which tend toward radiotherapy and away from surgery) and the importance of the cosmetic results; unlike the Americans, the French are concerned with the aesthetics of any form of treatment.[19] Characteristic of the American attitude toward cancer has been the need not only "to do something" but "to do it fast."[20] The American ethos influences how we practice medicine and in particular the need for action and aggressiveness in our response to cancer.

Western medicine in the United States is also affected in its practice by the particular moral ethos of the country. Most notable has been the emphasis upon personal autonomy. In *Democracy in America*, Alexis de Tocqueville observed that the social life made the people "form the habit of thinking of themselves in isolation and imagine their whole destiny is in their own hands."[21] Even in specialties that explicitly demonstrate the dependence patient's can have upon others, medicine has emphasized the "maximizing" of autonomy. Although in recent years there has been a call for communitarian values in bioethics,[22,23,24] this is a prophetic challenge that strives to counter the prevailing ethos of individualism. The ethos of individualism is expressed in many of the key terms of the contemporary medical ethics movement: advance directives, informed consent, decisional capacity, assisted suicide. Related to these ideas, there has arisen an expanded use of "rights" language in the United States to discuss moral issues.[25] Issues of end-of-life care have become a "right to die"; abortion is formulated as either a "right to choose" or a "right to life"; access to medical care is translated into a "right to health care."

The United States health care system is intimately tied to consumerism, a concept allied with notions of rights and autonomy. Although Anglos may believe that they have a right to select the type of health care they desire, many do not believe that there is a right to health care, unlike their northern neighbors in Canada. Access to health care in the United States is considered a principle of charity rather than a right by many. For them, health care is no less a commodity than other elements of life such as housing and food. The characteristics of allopathic medicine in the United States are summarized in Table 2.

Table 2: Characteristics of Allopathic Medicine in the United States

Positivistic
Mind-Body Dualistic
Person-Centered
Consumerist
Action-Oriented
Focused on Personal Autonomy

Our particular cultural assumptions also affect how we view illnesses such as cancer. In *Illness as Metaphor*, Susan Sontag argues that the West has understood various illnesses through metaphors that carry with them a moral import. Sontag observes that the "controlling metaphors" in the West's representation of cancer have been ones of warfare. When we describe a body with cancer, we use such words as "invasive" and "colonize," and we speak of medical treatment as "bombarded," "chemical warfare," and "killing cancer cells." This metaphoric language works both ways, she observes, in that we draw upon cancer itself as a metaphor for social problems. We speak, for example, of crime, communism, and terrorism as a "cancer" in the society that "spreads" throughout the social body. Sontag compares the adverse portrayals of cancer in Western art to the romantic ones of tuberculosis: "The dying tubercular is pictured as made more beautiful and more soulful; the person dying of cancer is portrayed as robbed of all capacities of self-transcendence, humiliated by fear and agony."[26] The stigma of cancer is perhaps best illustrated by the fear of even voicing the word. In *At the Will of the Body*, Arthur Frank, someone with the dubious distinction of having a heart attack and being diagnosed with cancer within two years, reflects that, "We do not call heart attack "h.a." Cancer alone is mythologized as some savage god, whose very name will invoke its presences."[27]

Breaking The Cultural Frame

The social scientists Gregory Bateson and Erving Goffman applied the concept of a "frame" to social situations; they argued that all social interactions are framed in ways that signal to the various participants how we are to understand what is going on.[28,29] For example, in order for someone to know that we are "joking" with them instead of insulting them, we use various signals in facial expressions and tone, and, if one misunderstands the our intentions, we can explicitly declare "I am just kidding you!" We can then quickly reframe the situation by stating, "Let me be serious for a moment." Deborah Tannen, a linguist, recommends that during periods when communication is difficult that we "break" the frame and talk about the difficulty we are having talking.[30] She believes that often miscommunication occurs when people have different signals. These signals are socially learned, and, Tannen suggests, we should, on occasion, expressly talk about the signals--what Bateson referred to as "metacommunication"--when we are having a difficulty conveying our ideas or feelings.

In a similar manner, health care professionals can break the cultural frame of an interaction by explicitly exploring the difficulty understanding the patient's cultural frame for communication. By making statements such as "in my culture we believe that," "I was raised to think," or "as a physician I tend to value," health care professionals are able to talk about the cultural frame of allopathic medicine to their patients. In breaking the cultural frame, a health care professional is also acknowledging the contingent nature of their beliefs. By admitting that one's ideas are not the only way of thinking, one licenses others to share their perspective. This type of self-conscious dialogue has been a standard technique social scientists have used to understand other cultures. Paul Rabinow argues that when an ethnographer engages a member of a community to explain something about that world a new "language" must be created.[31] When one breaks the cultural frame of an encounter with the patient, one does so by creating a temporary liminal language, which enables both to understand and be understood. Ethnographers, unlike health care professionals, normally have the luxury of time to construct this liminal language. Even in extended periods of fieldwork this shared language will create only a "partial and thin" understanding for the ethnographer, and health care professionals must make do with an even more tenuous understanding.

Making Translators Part Of The Team

As mentioned above, the use of intimates as translators should be considered only when one has first sought out professional translators and failed. Professional translators are, however, often misused. Some health care professionals treat translators as if they were language machines that simply dole out equivalent words and phrases. Health care professionals need to make translators feel that they are a part of the medical team or at the very least they are there to assist in reaching specific medical goals. Since communication entails more than merely words but also the body and an entire array of cultural signs, translators must be able to provide information that make the patient's statements intelligible to the health care professional and vice versa. Ideally such individuals should function more as cultural translators than language translators.

If one expects translators to provide assistance in the language and also to address cultural meanings and nuances of the medical problems, they can serve as important sources for cross-cultural understanding.   Translators should feel comfortable to indicate areas of the medical interview where there are potential conflicts or where particular styles of communication can indicate a vital cultural subtext.   One should always convene with translators prior to meeting with the patient so that one can quickly state the goals of this encounter and any concerns that one has about the patient.[32]   Translators should also be told that they are being depended upon to provide information that they think outsiders need in order to understand the patient's statements.   Afterwards there should be a short meeting between translator and the health care professional to allow them both to evaluate the encounter and to raise issues that need to be explored further.

TECHNIQUES FOR PREVENTION

Rather than responding to each new crisis, it is better to draw upon techniques that can anticipate problems. These techniques are best employed when one has a large and distinct ethnic population within your area.

Locate Cultural Informants

The concept of a cultural informant is borrowed from qualitative social science. An informant is a member of a community who assists the ethnographer in understanding the culture. Informants tend to be unusual people, who are able to act in a bridging fashion, so they need to have or acquire the kind of self-reflexivity mentioned above. The best informants generally are individuals on the social fringe of their culture. These socially marginalized individuals are often highly conscious of the cultural categories, for they themselves do not fit completely within them.

Ascertain the Community's Clinical Experience

Clinicians rely on their "clinical experience" to make sense of their problems. In a similar manner, community's have their own experiential knowledge in that they learn about medical problems through sharing narratives with each other. There is nothing unusual about this sharing of stories (it is a part of Anglo culture as well); communities (especially those who do not have members trained allopathically) draw upon each other's experiences in order to understand and predict how allopathic physicians will respond to particular situations. Not knowing these narratives can place a clinician at a disadvantage. Understanding, for example, that a previous family member has died of cancer may assist one in explaining how this instance of cancer is both like and different from the other family member's illness. Furthermore individuals may learn about cancer and the various medical treatments through other members of the community.   Some individuals who are recent immigrants to the United States or live in culturally isolated communities are often unfamiliar with what are considered reliable sources of information or are not fluent enough in the language to be able to understand information from such sources.

As with the Hmong family, there can be an entire array of other medical consultants who help make the diagnosis. A clinician needs to learn about these experiences and, when appropriate, revise the community's perceptions. In some communities, going to a physician is--for economic or cultural grounds--an act of last resort, and patients may elect to consult professional and non-professional healers within their community before coming to the allopathic system. Although it seems (as in the issue concerning this Hmong family) that allopathic medicine is viewed as a binary opposite to "alternative" or traditional forms of treatment, many people mix several forms of medical treatments. The recent movement in the United States to think of non-allopathic treatments as "complementary" rather than "alternative" mirrors how many people already conceive of these treatments. A clinician should whenever possible think of these other healers as colleagues rather than as competitors and be open to learning about their practices. One of the issues that was involved in the Hmong example is that the family saw the allopathic treatment as making their daughter sick (which was in some ways true) and did not trust that causing pain could in the end help their daughter. In order to prevent these conflicts health care professionals are obligated to learn the stories of the community: their religious, mythic, and paradigmatic ones and their particular experiences with allopathic medicine.

Identify Redressive Actions

When moral conflicts in many hospitals rise to a crisis level, health care professionals can call a meeting of an ethics committee. The concept of gathering together a group of individuals to discuss the problem and provide some recommendations seems to be a sensible way to deal with social conflict. Many cultural assumptions underlie this practice, assumptions that may not be shared by others.

The cultural anthropologist Victor Turner observed that within the life of a community that are periods of social tension or, what he termed, social dramas. Social life is not a stagnant entity but one awash in crisis and resolution. Turner discerned four phases in social dramas:[33,34]

> 1. Breach, in which there is a break in the normal social relations
> 2. Crisis, in which their is an escalation and people "take sides"
> 3. Redressive action, in which a formal structure comes forth to contain and resolve the problem
> 4. Reintegration, in which following the redressive action a resolution occurs and harmony restored.

A meeting of the ethics committee is one of the redressive actions that can take place within a hospital environment. These committee meetings are a part of the larger pattern of moral crisis management within the hospital environment.

Other communities have other means of resolving problems, means that do not necessarily entail a gathering together of individuals in a committee. Some communities contact a particular individual, as the traditional Jewish method of requesting the opinion of a rabbi, and some communities believe that one should turn directly to a divine entity for assistance. In the Hmong case, it was reported that the health care professionals should have contact the elders of the community. Obviously the redressive action of the court hearing was not recognized by the Hmong family. Consequently health care professionals should have a general understanding of the various redressive actions common within the community and how to work with these mechanisms in order to resolve moral conflicts.

ABIDING QUESTIONS

Morally and legally the United States has reached a consensus that competent adults have the right to refuse any medical treatment; the seemingly tragic outcome of some of these decisions are the anticipated consequences of a politically liberal society. This policy provides helpful guidance for resolving many moral conflicts, especially in problems that arise from cultural conflicts, but it can seem unworkable when health care professionals are faced with marginal cases.

Children And Adolescents

Perhaps the most difficult and contentious issues surround the care of minors. Like the case involving the Hmong family, such issues seem to bring into question our liberal concepts of respect for others and ask how far we are willing to honor the worldview of others. The prevailing response to this issue is that society has a responsibility to take custody temporarily away from the parents; this is justified by the claim that children have yet to "choose" the cultural beliefs of their parents and we do not know if as adults they will do so. There are a number of problems with this argument. First, what does it mean to choose a worldview? People can alter the worldview they were raised in but this usually entails a radical revision of their values. Second, even if people can choose a worldview and upon maturation people tended to reject the worldview of their upbringing, why should the default worldview be that of allopathic medicine? There is no way to argue rationally for the superiority of one worldview over another (otherwise we would have to accept that all other people in the world were irrational), so we must accept that the selection of allopathic medicine is a result of the political dominance of people who accept this worldview. If the majority of this culture were Hmong then perhaps Anglo parents would be forced to undergo shamanism. Third, forcing families to accept allopathic medicine can result in their reluctance to use the system when they believe that their control over the care of their children will be jeopardized.

Adolescents, of course, further complicate this issue, for they can sometiems demonstrate the intellectual and emotional maturity we expect to find in adults. The legal concept of a "mature minor" makes sense in such cases, and we should feel comfortable giving some adolescents the right to refuse (or accept) medical treatments that fit their personal religious or cultural perspectives.

The Cultural Catch-22

In a study of informed consent on a Navajo reservation, Joseph Carrese and Lorna Rhodes discovered that in the Navajo worldview a discussion of the potential risks of a medical treatment would make such events more likely to take place. Language, from the Navajo perspective, is not simply a mirror of the world but can alter reality. Informed consent as it has been traditionally practiced in American bioethics is thus viewed as a harmful practice.[35] The problem this raises is how do you inform a Navajo patient in order to determine if they wish to receive information? This creates a kind of cultural catch-22 that can be found in other areas of cross-cultural medicine. For example, it has been shown that some communities such as Italian-American do not believe that patients diagnosed with carcinoma should be informed of their illness or its prognosis.[36] Yet once again if such a belief is found to be culturally based how does one ask someone whether they wish to know if they have cancer? Although one could respond that one should discuss with patients about the future possibility of such a situation, once again this is a luxury of time and continuity of care that not all clinicians possess. Even then, how does one know that the patient who said that they did not wish to know several years ago still does not wish to know?

CONCLUSION

In this chapter some tools have been offered for assisting health care professionals in caring for people from different cultures. Although the initial impulse for many is for a simple list of beliefs and practices, we should be wary of this desire. It represents a need to place people in easily identifiable categories and sometimes this need can cause conflicts and tragic mistakes. Instead we should first become conscious of the cultural assumptions within our own healing practices; we need to identify how our own practices are part of larger cultural patterns (of language, worldview, values, and ethos), which seem to us "self-evident" and "natural." The techniques for resolution proposed in this chapter are rooted in this exercise of self-awareness. Once we are aware of this assumption, we can begin to find the parallel beliefs and practices of others. Through the assistance of translators and consultants we can acknowledge and on occasion break our cultural frames.

Acknowledgements: The author would like to thank Kathryn Montgomery and Joel Frader for reading earlier drafts of this paper.

REFERENCES

1. Vu T. "Laotian Teen Defies Court-Ordered Chemotherapy." 1994, National Public Radio/Morning Edition: Washington, D.C.

2. Herne HE, *et al.* The difference that culture can make in end-of-life decision making. Cambr Quar Hlthcare Ethics 1998;7: 27-40.

3. Lock, M. "Education and Self Reflection: Teaching about Culture, Health and Illness." In *Health and Cultures: Exploring the Relationships*, R. Masi et al., ed. Mosaic Press: Oakville, Ontario, 1993.

4. Lock 149.

5. Dixon JL, Smalley MG. Jehovah's witnesses: the surgical/ethical challenge. JAMA 1981;246:2471-2472.

6. Geertz C. *The Interpretation of Cultures.* New York: Basic Books, 1973, p 14.

7. Hall ET. *The Hidden Dimension. Garden* City: Anchor Books-Doubleday, 1966.

8. Argyle M. "Non-verbal Communication in Human Social Interaction." In *Non-Verbal Communication*, R.A. Hinde, ed. Cambridge: Cambridge University Press, 1972.

9. Myers GE, Myers MT. *The Dynamics of Human Communication.* 4th ed. New York: McGraw-Hill, 1985.

10. Geertz , p. 127.

11. Conquergood D, Thao P, Thao X. *I Am a Shaman: A Hmong Life Story with Ethnographic Commentary.* Minneapolis: University of Minnesota, 1989.

12. Capron AM. In Re Helga Wanglie. Hast Cent Rep 1991; (September-October): 26-28.

13. Wanning, E. *Culture shock!* Singapore: Time, 1991.

14. Lanier AR, Gay CW. *Living in the U.S.A.* 5th ed. Yarmouth, Maine: Intercultural Press, 1996.

15. Hunter KM. Narrative, literature, and the clinical exercise of practical reason. J Med Philos 1996; 21:303-320.

16. Hunter KM. *Doctors' Stories: The Narrative Structure of Medical Knowledge.* Princeton, New Jersey: Princeton University Press, 1991.

17. Kleinman A. *Writing at the Margin: Discourse Between Anthropology and Medicine.* Berkeley: University of California Press, 1995, p. 30.

18. Conquergood, Thao, Thao 58.

19. Payer L. *Medicine and Culture.* New York: Penguin, 1988, p. 53.

20. Payer, p. 137.

21. Quoted in: Fox RW, Kloppenberg JT, eds. *A Companion to American Thought.* Malden, Massachusetts: Blackwell, 1995, p. 337.

22. Kuczewski MG. *Casuistry and Its Communitarian Critics.* Kennedy Inst Ethics J 1994; 4, no. 2: 99-116.

23. MacIntyre, A. "The Return to Virtue Ethics." In *The Twenty-Fifth Anniversary of Vatican II: A Look Back and A Look Ahead.* R.E. Smith, ed.. Braintree, MA: The Pope John Center, 1990.

24. Emanuel EJ. *The Ends of Human Life.* Boston: Harvard University Press, 1991.

25. Glendon MA. *Rights Talk.* New York: Free Press, 1991.

26. Sontag S. *Illness as Metaphor and AIDS and Its Metaphors.* New York: Doubleday, 1990, p. 16.

27. Frank A. *At the Will of The Body.* Boston: Houghton , 1991, p. 97.

28. Bateson G. *Steps to an Ecology of Mind.* New York: Ballantine, 1972.

29. Goffman E. *Frame Analysis.* Cambridge: Harvard University Press, 1974.

30. Tannen D. *That's Not What I Meant!.* New York: Morrow, 1986.

31. Rabinow P. *Reflections on Fieldwork in Morocco.* Berkeley: University of California Press, 1977, p. 154-155.

32. Boston City Hospital. *The Bilingual Medical Interview.* Boston: Boston Area Health Education Center, 1991.

33. Turner V. *Dramas, Fields, and Metaphors: Symbolic Action in Human Society.* Ithaca: Cornell University Press, 1974.

34. Turner V. *Schism and Continuity in an African Society: A Study of Ndembu Village Life.* Manchester: Manchester University Press, 1957.

35. Carrese JA, Rhodes LA. Western bioethics on the Navajo reservation." JAMA 1995; 274:826-829.

36. Surbone A. Truth telling to the patient. JAMA 1992; 268:1661-1662.

4 RELIGIOUS/SPIRITUAL CONCERNS IN CARING FOR THE CANCER PATIENT

James F. Bresnahan, S.J., J.D., L.L.M., Ph.D.
John M. Merrill, M.D.

INTRODUCTION

Often, medical care givers fail to fully attend to religious and spiritual concerns of patients and instead assign responsibility elsewhere. It is frequently thought of as somebody else's job, such as that of the chaplain. Occasionally, a caregiver may take the initiative and inquire whether the patient would like to see one of the hospital's pastoral care team or some other religious minister of the patient's choice. But, given the secular and business-like milieu of medicine today, the religious and spiritual concerns of patients and their caregivers are often neglected as caregivers and patients focus on high technology diagnosis and treatment. Yet both patients and their caregivers bring the religious and moral convictions and commitments that have shaped their lives and actions to each clinical encounter.[1] In a situation of serious illness or injury, patients confront a crisis of meaning; they become aware of actual or anticipated loss of function, and with that, intimations of their mortality. It is normal, then, that they begin to reflect on what this illness or injury means to them. They find they have needs for some form of sharing their reflections and for supporting these reflections. Patients will often look to the medical caregiver to satisfy these needs.

When religious concerns are explicitly articulated by the patient, caregivers may be puzzled, even embarrassed, about how to deal with them. This is especially true when these concerns present an obstacle to the proposed treatment. In such a situation, clinicians are forced to realize that sincerely held beliefs and deep personal commitments play an important role, whether helpful or harmful, in achieving a good and clinically effective therapeutic relationship. Thus, clinicians must be adept at listening, and, as they listen, at integrating the background echoes of their own values and beliefs.

In order to promote this aspect of the therapeutic alliance, it seems worthwhile to consider some aspects of the religion-medical practice relationship. Serious forethought about the nature and impact of religious and spiritual concerns on medical decision making can aid caregivers to deal with this challenge in creative and effective ways. In general, we treasure the American tradition of freedom of religious belief, including freedom not to be religious in any traditional sense. Thoughtful and sympathetic inquiry based upon a reflection upon one's own deep convictions, can empower a dialog which will provide patients with a sense of being understood and liberated as they undergo medical diagnosis and treatment.

RELIGIOUS/SPIRITUAL CONCERNS IN THE CONTEMPORARY PLURALISTIC CONTEXT

It is important to remember that our contemporary North American clinical medical ethics (or bioethics) has developed within a morally and religiously pluralistic culture and society.[2] While religious thinkers have made important contributions to this development,[3] clinical medical ethics today encompasses a variety of competing views and claims about the normative content of moral obligation and ideal. This is most obvious in disputes about abortion, about physician assisted suicide, and generally also about matters of sexuality and fertility promotion or control. At best, the holders of these competing views are in civil conversation with each other.[4] Only very rarely does one find unanimously accepted moral values or principles or maxims, at least on the abstract theoretical level.

On the other hand, where the civil conversation is carried on by those who disagree, they are empowered to explore thoughtfully together the concrete ethical problems, and so they can succeed, together, in finding practical ways to cooperate in caring for patients and their families.[5] This suggests that the experience of those engaged in ecumenical discourse between churches and religions may provide some help to medical caregivers in their efforts to be creative and effective in dealing with religious and spiritual concerns not only of their colleagues but also of their patients.

It should be noted that contemporary moral and religious pluralism of viewpoints with which patients and caregivers must deal is presented not only in matters which most persons would readily recognize as explicitly "religious"--matters concerning what some call "faith" or "belief in a higher power." (In that sense, the "religious" is usually linked to an historic shared community of belief--one of the "world religions" in one of each particular religion's various forms or sects). This pluralism is also very much present in what others might assert not to be at all "religious"-- their attitude of skepticism about (agnosticism) or denial of (atheism) any such "higher power." (Such an outlook is often more individualistic than communitarian, though it may be derive also from such contemporary communities of conviction as "ethical humanism"). The point is that whether or not overtly religious in the usual sense, deeply held moral convictions and commitments involve the particular person's profound sense of personal moral integrity, and such convictions and commitments are bound to find expression in matters crucial to the person's sense of personal integrity. An ecumenical conversation tries to respect this. A similar effort can be made by the medical caregiver to respect patients' spiritual and religious concerns

The origins of religious and spiritual concerns need to be appreciated, too. In time of crisis, a search for meaning in one's human living and dying is generally experienced and acknowledged by most people. This phenomenon becomes more explicit and influential in times of crisis such as illness or injury, and in facing one's dying. Philosophers and theologians, of course, describe and evaluate this phenomenon of self-experience in many different ways. One individual may consider it an aberration and resolutely refuse to entertain thoughts about it. Another may explore it as a matter of "personal philosophy of life," while many acknowledge it to be a "religious" search in a more traditional sense.

The Protestant theologian, Paul Tillich, offers a helpful way to look at this experience of search for meaning in time of crisis. He classifies as "religious" all forms of profound personal moral concern and commitment which arise out of this search for meaning; he calls such commitment "religious" in the sense that the search for meaning and its outcome in a personal moral stance focuses on matters of what he calls "ultimate concern."[6] This formulation of Tillich's has been used by the United States Supreme Court in interpreting the scope of federal statutes which recognize "conscientious objection" to participation in war. Such a conscientious stance is said to arise out of "religious conviction" when it includes "what you take seriously without any reservation" even if this does not involve explicit reference to a "supreme being."[7]

So, moral concern and commitment involving ultimate personal loyalties in which an individual finds expressed the deepest meaning of life and moral decision-making lead that person to try to embody them in practice in order to achieve and maintain a basic "personal integrity". Obviously, any religious and spiritual conviction and commitment understood broadly in this way can strongly influence the thinking and so the participation in decision-making of cancer patients in their awareness of an impending personal crisis. It can also influence caregivers, given its impact within their sense of professional commitment, though this may not always be explicitly acknowledged by them.

RELIGIOUS OR SPIRITUAL CONCERNS AND THERAPEUTIC ALLIANCE

In what follows, however, no claim is made that one must attend to any particular religious concerns or commitments, whether of patients or of caregivers, because such religious concerns are simply identical with the normative content of some purportedly universally recognized normative medical ethical obligation to which all must submit. Such will not be found today in our pluralist culture. Rather, a pragmatic (but not basely opportunistic) claim is advanced here: if caregivers want to strive to achieve a clinically successful therapeutic alliance with their patients, they cannot ignore the religious and spiritual concerns of all parties in the medical decision-making process. Caregivers must take careful cognizance of, and then deal creatively with, these important concerns.

Explicit, empathetic but critical, attention to such religious and spiritual concerns may support and enhance the development of this therapeutic relationship and can even affect its outcome. This attentiveness is most of all needed when religious/spiritual convictions and commitments produce conflict and misunderstanding which undermine efforts to achieve medically urgent goals. The capacity of the clinician to listen to and really hear what the patient means is crucial. If in the particular medical interaction between patient and caregivers, all parties are satisfied that their deepest moral and religious convictions have been identified, understood, and, as far as humanly possible, respected, an effective therapeutic alliance will be formed and often enhanced. It seems likely, as well, that the effort to achieve this effective therapeutic alliance may even contribute to the technical success of the medical interaction (consider the placebo effect of a good healer-patient relationship).

It is commonly affirmed in contemporary ethics of care-giving that clinicians must strive to achieve not only accurate diagnosis and appropriate planning of therapeutic interventions but also, as far as possible, an empathetic, indeed compassionate, understanding of each patient's personal situation and needs.[8] Caregivers make this effort in order to be able adequately and effectively to inform the patient and to obtain the patient's uncoerced consent and cooperation. They try to avoid both coercion and seduction[9] of their patients in proposing therapy. These are fundamental aspects of an effective therapeutic alliance, and attentiveness to religious and spiritual concerns can be seen as a dimension of these expectations and ideals.

ACHIEVING THERAPEUTIC ALLIANCE BETWEEN THE CANCER PATIENT AND THE CAREGIVER

When a patient is diagnosed with cancer, the clinician can expect that the patient is undergoing a particularly profound personal sense of crisis. Within a culture in which cancer is a deeply feared diagnosis, for many almost a death sentence, the cancer patient anticipates not only loss of function and the suffering of distressing treatments, but also the potential loss of life itself. The cancer patient is in crisis, rendered vulnerable, perhaps disoriented and desperate. An emotional roller coaster ride begins to produce highs and lows in the midst of which the patient looks to religious and spiritual roots (in the wide sense already noted above) for balance and solace.

The caregiver dealing with the cancer patient must take account of this, fully. Confronted with the patient's experience of crisis, the caregiver should expect to be challenged to support the patient through varying, at times extreme, emotional reactions and to encounter explicit expression of the patient's religious and spiritual beliefs and commitments, or other puzzling reactions which may conceal religious or spiritual concerns. Thus, as patients and caregivers interact with each other through a series of diagnostic and therapeutic interventions, they will confront a variety of reactions to remission or progression of disease which provoke explicit dialog about these spiritual and religious concerns.

Eventually, the caregiver will frequently have to discuss with a cancer patient why a decision needs to be made whether to continue cure-oriented treatment or instead palliative measures aimed primarily at relief of suffering.[10]   Here the religious/spiritual beliefs and commitments of each patient interact powerfully with those of the caregiver, sometimes in ways that support their cooperation, at other times in ways that disrupt their relationship and undermine clinical medical success.

The cancer patient may find courage for submitting to the rigors of chemotherapy, radiation therapy, or surgery from religious beliefs and commitments. Clinicians will want to encourage this even explicitly, but only to the extent that caregivers can do that without violation of their own deeply personal commitments. In acting out his or her beliefs and commitments, the patient may in other circumstances oppose a recommended course of treatment; even become "non-compliant," in ways that are, for the clinicians, puzzling and distressing. Caregivers need to prepare themselves to understand, as thoroughly and empathetically as they are able, how particular religious and spiritual commitments of each patient shape these very different responses. This empathetic approach is especially challenging if the caregivers cannot share the patient's commitments or even disagree heartily with them.

Hope as a Support or as Source of Disruption in the Care of the Cancer Patient

Hope frequently appears as an expression of the religious or spiritual outlook and commitment of a patient. If inspired by religious faith, one's hope may sometimes express a confidence in God's loving providential care of the person, in the vicissitudes of this life, and in the next life as well. Sometimes hope reflects less high theology, but rather an expectation of cure that borders on a superstitious attempt to control hidden powers. Alternatively, hope may take the form of a kind of agnostic or atheistic stoic realism. Each particular patient's hope is shaped partly by that person's faith in God and divine providence, or trust in hidden powers, or in the need for a stoic realism. In addition, each person's hope is also shaped, in part at least, by what the caregiver leads the patient to understand and believe about the disease process and about both the realistic possibilities and the limits of medical response to it. A mutual conditioning process is at work through which the religious and spiritual attitudes of the patient are shaped by what the clinician seeks to communicate to the patient as medical information or recommendation.

Because of the influence the clinician can have on a patient's hope, the clinician must inquire about what the patient hopes for, and why. Does the patient expect divine intervention to prevent suffering and death, or to sustain the patient through possible suffering and dying? Does the patient expect something like divine powers from the technical expertise of the caregiver and the mysterious efficacy of high technology and pharmacology? Especially with regard to recognizing the limits as well as the possibilities of medical treatment, has the caregiver helped the patient to be realistic in their hopes, or has the caregiver encouraged "false hope"?

Hope goes beyond a desire for something to be given. Hope carries some expectation of what will come to be. For cancer patients, hope is challenged by a deterioration in their health status. Recently Simonton[11] and Siegel[12] have agreed that, in the face of medical uncertainty, there is nothing wrong with hope. Quill quotes a dying patient saying: "There is a world of difference between no hope and a ray of hope! It's black and white, night and day."[13]

How varied are the meanings given to hope. With a realistic hope, patients can accept a particular diagnosis and remain at peace with an uncertain prognosis. But, where there may be a great difference between a ray of hope and no hope, from the point of view of the caregiver and the patient, there is an even more radical difference between hope that is realistic about limits of the power of medicine and of the clinician, and false hope.

A factor in the caregiver's share in shaping the patient's hope is the amount of time it takes for the clinician to understand the particular patient well enough to impart effectively some idea of what can realistically be hoped for. On the one hand, a "ray of hope" may be given to the patient by a clinician that suggests an additional chemotherapy with the words, "there may be this one, last chance." But, that sentence may also leave the patient fearful, not daring to ask further questions or raise doubts, confused about how now to hope. A clinician would need far more time to explain why there is really "no hope" for improvement in the disease--but also why there is solid grounding for a realistic hope in what the clinician can do and intends to do in the face of this devastating news. The healing possibilities offered by palliative care and the promise of continued presence of the caregiver could enliven a hope where cure of disease can no longer be hoped for.

To engender "false hope," however, when the true nature of the patient's situation finally becomes apparent, too often devastates the patient, and does more harm than that produced by an effort to help the patient have realistic hopes. When a manifestly false hope crashes, there ensues for the patient a sustained sense of betrayal by the caregiver. This can diminish, if not utterly destroy, the effectiveness of the healing relationship between them. This can even impair the possibilities of technical success of treatment (now distrust undermines potential benefit from the placebo effect).

Pondering the complexity of hope confirms a need for some serious forethought and reflection by clinicians. The way in which each clinician's own deeply held moral beliefs and commitments can come into play in dialog about the patient's religious and spiritual concerns must be considered in order for an effective therapeutic alliance between caregiver and patient to develop.

THE CAREGIVER'S NEED FOR SELF-AWARENESS

Clinicians working with cancer patients face not only the technical challenge to their medical competence but also the particularly demanding challenge of achieving sympathetic insight and responsiveness to their patients' religious and spiritual concerns. The most basic requirement for meeting this challenge is that clinicians accept the ancient injunction, "know thyself." This involves not only learning to listen to the patient but, above all, clinicians must engage in honest self-assessment about their own beliefs and deepest moral convictions. Clinicians must consider how these beliefs and convictions shape their propensity to respond in certain ways to different, even conflicting, religious and spiritual concerns of patients. What causes a clinician to encourage or oppose certain patients as they react to crisis out of religious or spiritual (in the broad sense) concerns? Why does one react so, and how can one try to manage these reactions creatively for the benefit of patients in a way that does not compromise but rather sustains one's own deep sense of personal and professional integrity?

Such efforts at honest self-assessment and self-knowledge need not be feared. The experience of ecumenical religious conversation testifies that one is never required simply to capitulate to religious or spiritual convictions of others when these convictions contradict one's own deepest loyalties. Medical caregivers should not become "hired guns" who do always just what a patient demands. Where one encounters disagreement so fundamental that no reasonable grounds of cooperation can be discerned, the clinician can and should be ready to help the patient to find other caregivers with whom a better therapeutic alliance can be achieved. Before one takes that ultimate step, however, understanding one's own religious and spiritual convictions and commitments may provide insight into what patients are experiencing and why, and about what kinds of cooperation one can achieve with patients with whom one differs, even radically. Realizing the boundaries that one's own deepest concerns put upon the therapeutic alliance can be a source for discovering possibilities for understanding, how the other sees and reacts to the problem that clinician and patient seek to deal with together. Steven H. Miles has related how he was able to find ways to cooperate with persons with whom he disagreed; maintaining as a doctor the continuing trust of a dying patient's family who were opposing his and others' efforts to obtain a court order to permit them to terminate the patient's ventilator support.[14] Practical ways to cooperate can often be found in spite of deep disagreements.

With effort at personal reflection and self-knowledge, caregivers will find that every instance of conflict between patient and caregiver, in matters of religious and spiritual concern, no matter how difficult and stressful, can become a source of renewed insight and deeper understanding of the forms in which such concerns affect both self and others. The clinician who accepts the challenge to develop personal insight and is open to understanding others can be encouraged by the realization that the journey of self-awareness is a worthwhile one. There are no ready-made formulas for resolving once and for all, conflicts among deeply personal aspects of the clinician-patient encounter. Experience supports insight; appropriate understanding empowers creative compassionate response.

CONCLUSION

Maxims to help each clinician may well be formed in the course of this on-going experience, but these usually will be temporary aids to diagnosis and resolution of the problems encountered in shaping creative responses to religious and spiritual concerns of patients and families. Such practical maxims will need to be further refined and revised as each one's experience and insight develops. This studied openness to one's own experience in coping with the religious and spiritual concerns of self and others, combined with imaginativeness in seeking resolution of conflicts and maximizing effectiveness of cooperation, will be most effective to prepare the clinician for the challenge of dealing well with the religious and spiritual concerns of patients in crisis.

What can and should be expected from this effort is that one's search for self-knowledge in matters of deep conscientious conviction will protect the caregiver from habits of unwitting arrogance when responding to those religious and spiritual concerns of patients, even if these concerns seem irritating to or obstructive of what one believes professional duty and excellence demand. Indeed, this search can also often lead to a comforting sense of gratitude for benefits that, the effort to deal well with the religious and spiritual concerns of patients will produce in the course of the healing relationship between caregiver and patient.

REFERENCES

1. Bresnahan, James F. "Death: II. Contemporary Art of Dying." in *Encyclopedia of Bioethics,* Rev. ed. Warren Thomas Reich, ed. New York: Simon & Schuster Macmillan, 1995, vol. I, 551-54. See also, Bresnahan JF. The Catholic art of dying. America 1995;173 (#14):12-16.

2. Lovin, Robin W. "Ethics: V. Religion and Morality," in *Encyclopedia of Bioethics,* Rev. ed. Warren Thomas Reich, ed. New York: Simon & Schuster Macmillan, 1995, vol. II, 758-64.

3. Gustafson JM. *The Contributions of Theology to Medical Ethics.* Milwaukee: Marquette U. Press, 1975.

4. Engelhardt HT. *The Foundations of Bioethics.* 2nd ed., New York: Oxford U. Press, 1996.

5. Bresnahan, James F. "Ethical Dilemmas in Critical Care Medicine." in *Case Studies in Critical Care Medicine,* 2nd ed., Roy D. Cane, et al., eds. Chicago: Year Book Medical Publishers, 1991. See also, Jonsen, Albert R. "Casuistry." in *Encyclopedia of Bioethics,* vol. I, 344-50.

6. Tillich, Paul. *Shaking the Foundations.* New York: C. Scribners Sons, 1948.

7. United States v. Seeger, 380 U.S. 163, 35 Supr. Ct. Rep. 850 (1965), Opinion of Mr. Justice Clark and Concurring opinion of Mr. Justice Douglas.

8. Lustig, Andrew. "Compassion." in *Encyclopedia of Bioethics,* vol. I, 441-45. See also, Reich, Warren Thomas. "Care: I. History of the Notion of Care." and "Care: II. Historical Dimensions of an Ethic of Care." in *Encyclopedia of Bioethics,* vol. I, 319-36; and Jecker, Nancy S. & Reich, Warren Thomas. "Care: III. Contemporary Ethics of Care." in *Encyclopedia of Bioethics* vol I, 336-44.

9. Krant MJ. Rights of the cancer patient. CA 1975;25: 3-4.

10. Cassell E. *The Nature of Suffering and the Goals of Medicine.* New York: Oxford U. Press, 1991.

11. Simonton OC, et al., *Getting Well Again.* Los Angeles: Tarcher Publishing, 1978.

12. Siegel BS. *Love, Medicine & Miracles.* New York: Harper & Row, 1986.

13. Quill TE. *A Midwife through the Dying Process.* Baltimore: Johns Hopkins Press, 1996.

14. Miles SH. Interpersonal issues in the Wanglie case. Kennedy Inst Ethics J 1992;2: 61-72.

5 ARE THERE LIMITS TO ONCOLOGY CARE? (FUTILITY)

Gary R. Shapiro, M.D.

INTRODUCTION

Just when it looked like we had finally decided that patients were in charge, doctors and patients are again at odds over just "whose life it is anyway." Not long ago it was the patients and their families taking the doctors and their hospitals to court for the right to have unwanted life support withdrawn.[1] Now it seems that the tables have turned. It is the doctors and their hospitals who are going to court[2,3,4,5,6] to "deal... with families who demand inappropriate medical treatment for moribund patients."[7]

Death is no stranger to the cancer clinic. End-of-life concerns are the constant backdrop in front of which cancer doctors and cancer patients make treatment decisions.[8] Although oncologists face these ethical dilemmas every day, surprisingly few cancer journals deal with end-of-life issues in their publications.[9] This is particularly true when it comes to discussions of "futility." The concept of futility entered the medical literature in the late 1980s,[10,11,12] and it is now the subject of one in six articles devoted to medical ethics. Though the number of publications dealing with futility has doubled since the 1980s, fewer than 1% are in cancer journals.[13]

Oncologists don't do themselves or their patients any favors when they sit out the futility debate. These discussions often assume that most anticancer therapy is futile,[14] and cite a diagnosis of cancer as sufficient justification to withhold or withdraw life-prolonging therapy.[10,15] Futility claims may justify policies that categorically limit access to certain cancer care.[16]

Armed with ethical analyses about a doctor's duty,[17] outcomes' data,[18,19] and the latest policy statements,[20,21] doctors have raised the flag of futility with great passion. In their attempts to defend the profession, many doctors have forgotten that the doctor patient relationship is based on dialogue and education. Specific treatment decisions should be the natural conclusion of this dialogue not its beginning. Acceptable decisions regarding cancer treatment can be reached when attainable goals and patients' wishes are clearly identified.

THE ILLUSION OF FUTILITY: QUANTITATIVE/QUALITATIVE AND PHYSIOLOGIC STANDARDS

Through all the years of debate, resuscitation of the cancer patient has served as a standard case for advocates of medical futility. Citing the zero per cent discharge rate of resuscitated patients with metastatic cancer in Bedell's 1983 study,[22] Leslie Blackhall was among the first to use this argument against the practice of resuscitating patients with cancer.[10] Some years later, Kathy Faber-Langendoen also grounded her very similar conclusions in the concept of "quantitative" futility.[15]

Two different standards have emerged for doctors to use to determine when a particular treatment is futile. Lawrence Schneiderman and his colleagues advocate that a treatment should be considered futile when it has proven useless in the last 100 cases ("Quantitative Futility"); or when it merely preserves permanent unconsciousness, or cannot end dependence on intensive medical care ("Qualitative Futility").[23,24] On the other hand, Robert Truog and his colleagues accord the concept a very narrow role in medical decision making. By this restrictive standard, futility is limited to cases where a treatment cannot sustain physiologic life or it cannot achieve a desired physiologic effect.[25]

A report from Memorial Sloan-Kettering that appeared in the Journal of Clinical Oncology one month before the Faber-Langendoen review, readily demonstrates the problem with these types of analyses. This report showed a 10% discharge rate in the group of patients who had metastatic cancer. This compared favorably to resuscitated patients with non-cancer diagnoses.[26]

As though she were anticipating the Memorial Sloan-Kettering report, Blackhall buttresses her case with an argument from "qualitative" futility: "Furthermore… there are risks involved…including the development of a chronic vegetative state - which many believe is worse than death - or…survival after the initial resuscitation but with death occurring after an indefinite stay in the (ICU)."[10] The likelihood of either of these calamitous events occurring in a patient with advanced cancer is extremely low. Rational patients might just take the gamble.

Although the "physiologic" standard of futility makes fewer value judgments than either the "quantitative" or "qualitative" standard, it has become increasingly clear that no definition of futility is value free.[27] Indeed, studies[28,29] have confirmed that the multiple, often contradictory, ways doctors use "futility" usually support value judgments based on quality of life considerations. "Futility" is no less illusionary today than it was ten years ago.[12] It remains an elusive concept that is wielded as a "trump card" by doctors who believe that they know what is best for their patients.

PATERNALISM VS. INFORMED-CONSENT

In his 1995 essay,[30] Bruce Zawacki correctly identifies paternalism and informed-consent as the two ethical concepts that have come to be competing paradigms in the futility debate. Paternalism has a long history in medical decision making.[31] Although codes of medical ethics[32] no longer encourage doctors to act paternalistically toward their patients, arguments over paternalism continue to be at the heart of most moral problems in medicine. Doctors who once believed that they were supposed to act paternalistically toward their patients, are now told that they should never act paternalistically. Paternalism is not always wrong, and it is no wonder that such dogmatism has led doctors to develop the concept of "medical futility" to take "precedence over patient autonomy and permit... physicians to withhold or withdraw care deemed to be inappropriate without subjecting such a decision to patient approval."[30]

Informed consent is one of the cornerstones of medical ethics. Doctors have a moral[33] duty to provide their patients with comprehensible adequate information concerning any suggested treatment. A physician may not coerce a patient into consenting, and the physician must disclose to the patient the nature of the intervention, its risks and benefits, as well as the alternatives with their risks and benefits.[34] Given this information, rational patients may vary among themselves with regard to how they rank the harms and benefits of a suggested treatment. Although there are many clinical situations in which patients face only one rational choice, there are also a great many situations that permit more than one rational choice. On the other hand, "informed consent does not mean that patients can insist upon anything they might want. Rather, it is a choice among available..." and medically accepted treatment options."[35]

MEDICAL TREATMENT

The Theoretical Sense

In the theoretical sense a given intervention is considered a treatment for a malady[36] or a symptom only if it has, by some specific function inherent to that intervention, a capacity to eliminate, relieve, or prevent the harm caused by that malady or symptom.

For example, penicillin is a treatment for pneumococcal pneumonia because it has certain inherent qualities that make it efficacious against pneumococci. On the other hand, penicillin is not a treatment for herpes simplex virus because it lacks an inherent capacity to meet the goal of treatment: elimination, relief, or prevention of any of the harms caused by the herpes simplex virus infection. Other examples include Laetrile or coffee ground enemas for Hodgkin's Disease, and ampicillin for meningitis caused by an ampicillin-resistant strain of haemophilus influenza.

The Common Medical Sense

Our common use of the word treatment contains a qualification that is not given in the theoretical definition provided above. In this more common medical sense of the word, an intervention is considered a treatment for a malady or a symptom if by some specific function inherent to that intervention it will eliminate, relieve, or prevent the harm caused by that malady or symptom and it does not inherently (irrespective of any particular patient) involve unacceptable medical side effects.

Penicillin is also a treatment for pneumococcal pneumonia in this sense, because it has a high probability of meeting the goal of eliminating the harms caused by a pneumococcal infection. This outweighs the harms that might be caused by any one of a number of adverse side effects listed on the package insert.

On the other hand, though the therapeutic goal of removing a plantar wart can be achieved by a below the knee amputation (and amputation is therefore theoretically treatment for plantar warts), amputation is not considered medically to be a treatment for plantar warts; the harm caused by this "treatment" far outweighs any harm that is relieved by removing the wart in this manner. Radiation therapy for acne, chloramphenicol for streptococcal pharyngitis, and thalidomide for morning sickness are just a few of the long list of interventions that are treatments in the theoretical sense, but not treatments in the more common medical sense.

Medically Acceptable Treatment

For a medical intervention to be a medically acceptable treatment it must not only be a treatment in the common medical sense, but it must also be appropriate for the particular patient being treated. Penicillin may be a medically acceptable treatment for one patient with pneumococcal pneumonia, but it is certainly not a medically acceptable treatment for a patient who has a history of anaphylaxis to penicillin. The medical acceptability of a treatment is determined by the inherent qualities of the medical intervention as they relate to the unique nature of the individual patient.

A medical intervention is not medically acceptable treatment if: (A) for the specific patient being treated it results in harms indisputably greater than those harms eliminated, relieved, or prevented, or if (B) it is unable to meet its therapeutic goal for that specific patient.

Examples of the former situation are, the use of intravenous Heparin in a patient suffering from an acute deep venous thrombosis with a bleeding ulcer; and the case of the patient with the penicillin allergy referred to earlier. The latter situation is exemplified by the case of a patient who also has an acute deep venous thrombosis, but who, in this case, has an anti-thrombin III factor deficiency that makes Heparin an ineffective drug in his body.

Therefore, a medically acceptable treatment may be defined as a medical intervention that, for a particular patient, has a reasonable probability of eliminating, relieving, or preventing the specific harm(s) for which the treatment was intended without causing the patient some other harm (death, pain, disability, loss of freedom, or loss of pleasure[37]) that is <u>indisputably</u> greater than the harm eliminated, relieved, or prevented. What constitutes "reasonable" is of course open to debate, but we can state that at a bare minimum there must be some probability ("at least a modicum of potential benefit"[38]) of meeting the therapeutic goal considering both the nature of the treatment and the nature of the patient.

Desirable Medical Treatment

Even when all of the resources necessary to carry out a medically acceptable treatment are available, a medically acceptable treatment may still not be given to a patient if he does not desire it.[39,40] A patient's decision that certain goals are not worth pursuing is best seen as an assertion of personal values (ranking the harms caused by the treatment greater than the harms prevented) rather than of futility.

It is essential to recognize that any decision to provide a treatment to a patient depends upon two features. The establishment of medical acceptability is the necessary component, but this alone is not sufficient to lead one to subject the patient to the treatment. One must also take into account all of the modifying non-medical features. These include, but are not limited to, familial, racial,[33] ethnic,[41] fiscal, and social concerns. Of the non-medical features none is more important than how the patient ranks the harms involved.

However important such non-medical concerns may be in determining how desirable a medically acceptable treatment is, it is necessarily conditional upon the efficacy of the treatments primary function vis-à-vis the specific harms to be eliminated, relieved, or prevented.

In this light we can see that there is no conflict between what constitutes the patient's role in the decision making process and the doctor's prerogative. Therapeutic decisions are purely medical when there is no question about the harms or their ranking. If however, the ranking of harms is disputable, the patient's input is morally required. In other words, the only value decisions that doctors should make without consulting the patient are those where there is no rational disagreement. Clearly, these cases are exceedingly rare.

A DOCTOR'S DUTY

Except in emergencies, a physician has no duty to achieve the best consequences for his competent patients. Consent (or refusal) to a particular treatment is ultimately the sole prerogative of the patient,[42] but the ideal of shared decision making requires physicians to ensure that their patients are well informed. Abiding by a patient's values does not mean that a doctor should passively accept irrational choices or decisions that are unreasonable given the patient's ranking of the harms and benefits involved.[43] When a doctor guides a patient toward the treatment option that is most in keeping with the patient's ranking of harms and benefits, he is truly fulfilling his duty toward his patient. This is not unjustified paternalism.[44]

IRRATIONAL AND UNREASONABLE DECISIONS

Rational persons usually have no desire to consider ineffective treatments as viable alternatives, and a physician has no duty to inform patients about treatment options that are not medically acceptable. Acting rationally requires only not acting irrationally. A patient (or his family) acts irrationally when he acts in a way that he knows, or should know, will significantly increase the probability that he, or those he cares for, will suffer death, pain, disability, loss of freedom or loss of pleasure; and he does not have an adequate reason for so acting. An adequate reason is a conscious rational belief that can make doing what would otherwise be an irrational action rational. Such beliefs will always involve, either directly or indirectly, a belief that someone (oneself or others) will avoid a harm (death, pain, disability, loss of freedom, loss of pleasure) or gain a good (ability, freedom, or pleasure).[45]

A Rationally Allowed Decision

This analysis explains the behavior of an elderly Russian immigrant patient whom I took care of several years ago. Days before he was likely to die of metastatic pancreatic cancer he asked me to cancel his long standing Do Not Resuscitate order (DNR). This seemed like an irrational decision until he explained that he wanted to suspend the DNR order just long enough for his daughter to have a chance to see him. After fifteen years of separation, she was due to arrive from Moscow the following day. By ranking the pleasure that she would derive from the opportunity to see him one last time (even if he was unresponsive and on a ventilator) higher than the harm that would come to him from such a resuscitation attempt, he had an adequate reason for what would otherwise be an irrational action. With my help, he also decided to have the ventilator stopped within 24 hours of his daughter's visit, in the event that a successful resuscitation left him ventilator dependent.

The final point is especially important. Cancer patient's and their doctors usually know each other quite well, and, therefore, have the unique opportunity to develop this type of preventive ethics approach.[46] This approach includes, but is not limited to making Advance Directives.

This example also illustrates the importance of doctor-patient communication regarding the goals of treatment and the ranking of harms and benefits. Neither Schneiderman's "qualitative" or "quantitative" standards, nor Truog's "physiologic" standard explain why this patient's decision was rationally allowed. Both of these futility standards fail because they focus on outcome and not on process.

Though I would allow everyone in a similar position to make a similar decision, some may argue that such public advocacy would have harmful results. One such outcome could be the demoralizing effect that this type of decision might have on the medical and nursing staff required to participate in what they view as a "futile" endeavor.[47] Despite admonitions to the contrary,[48,49] concerns over bad financial outcomes and the utilization of scarce medical resources have been associated with the futility debate since it began. These concerns must be taken seriously, but they have no place at the bedside. They properly belong to those concerned with the formulation of public policy and legislative consensus.[50]

UNDERSTANDING THE BENEFITS AND HARMS OF TREATMENT

We have seen how pronouncements of futility serve to mask paternalism or prejudice, and excuse bedside rationing. Ultimately the appropriateness of a particular medical treatment is determined by how the patient ranks the benefits and harms.

Leukemia In An Octogenarian

Two years ago an 86 year old man presented to our hospital with acute myelogenous leukemia. The previous year an article appeared in the British Journal of Haematology reporting the outcome of acute myelogenous leukemia in patients aged 80 years and above. The journal article concluded "that currently available therapy cannot be recommended for patients aged 80 and over."[51] The harms of this expensive treatment were clear: certain loss of freedom and pleasure; a high probability of pain, disability, and even death. Weighing the evidence he concluded that, as awful as the harms of treatment were, there were no harms greater than the certainty of death from leukemia within the weeks to come. The 86 year old man is now 88, in complete remission, enjoying his family, and running his business.

With the benefit of hindsight, it is certainly hard to argue that induction chemotherapy for this gentleman was futile, and that this "natural-end cancer"[52] should have been allowed to bring him a peaceful death to close his long and fulfilling life. Even those who argue for the "compression of morbidity"[53] (a shorter period of illness prior to death in old age) as a method of saving dollars, would be hard pressed to balance the books against this factory owner.

Critics will maintain that exceptional cases like this should not be used to make policy decisions, but it is just such bedside cases that expose the conflict of values that underlie all discussions of futility. Society has the duty to make rational decisions to allocate medical resources, contain costs, and balance medical needs against other social concerns. Good public policy is made by facing these hard issues straight on, not by obscuring them under the rubric of futility.

Trade-Offs: Survival vs. Quality of Life

Although this patient's outcome was unusual, his decision making was not. Contrary to the opinion of most medical professionals, many patients are willing to accept severe toxicity from treatment for the small chance of extended life.[54] Even cancer chemotherapy patients are generally unwilling to trade-off survival rate for improved quality of life.[55] This is particularly true of the very old.[56]

Doctors frequently decide to withhold life-sustaining treatments from seriously ill patients. A recent SUPPORT report[57] eloquently demonstrates how physicians' tendency to underestimate elderly patients' desire for aggressive treatments results in high rates of withholding CPR (cardiopulmonary resuscitation), and other life-sustaining treatments.

Levels of Evidence

Most cancer patients want to actively participate in decision making with their doctors.[58] Assessments regarding the likelihood of a particular medical intervention meeting its therapeutic goal are essential components of the decision making process. These assessments are subject to the scientific method, and can be classified into three grades depending on their supporting levels of evidence. Grade A and B recommendations are those supported by level I (large randomized clinical trials with clear-cut results) and level II (small randomized clinical trials with uncertain results) evidence, respectively. Grade C recommendations are based on evidence from levels III (nonrandomized, concurrent cohort comparisons), IV (nonrandomized, historical cohort comparisons), or V (case series without controls).[59]

Classification of Medical Interventions

Sharpe and Faden[60] have shown how these Grades of Evidence bring comprehensible, adequate information to the process of informed consent. By correlating the level of evidence with the preponderance of anticipated harms and benefits, their system helps us understand how doctors make recommendations regarding the medical appropriateness of treatment, and how patients can then make rational decisions regarding the desirability of treatment based on their own values.

Possibly Beneficial

These interventions are thought to be preponderantly beneficial, but only on the basis of weak, Grade C evidence. Radical prostatectomy for well-differentiated, localized prostate cancer in patients less than 75 years old would fit into this category.

Indicated and Highly Indicated

These interventions are also thought to be preponderantly beneficial, but, unlike the previous category, the evidence (Grade B and A, respectively) supporting their efficacy is strong (Indicated) or definitive (Highly Indicated). Examples in these categories are adjuvant chemotherapy regimens for women with lymph node positive breast cancer.

Possibly Harmful

These interventions are thought to be preponderantly harmful based on only anecdotal evidence, case reports, or uncontrolled studies (Grade C). Many second-line chemotherapy protocols for metastatic non-small cell lung cancer fall into this group.

Equivocal

The ratio of benefit to harm is roughly the same in these interventions that are also supported by weak levels of evidence (Grade C). The use of adjuvant chemotherapy in stage II colon cancer is in this category.

Contraindicated

Good evidence (Grade A or B) is sufficiently to place these preponderantly harmful interventions outside of medically acceptable care. Laetrile and adjuvant chemotherapy for gastric cancer are both examples of interventions that are not medically acceptable.

Non-indicated

When good evidence (Grade A or B) establishes that the benefit/harm ration is roughly equivalent, treatments are generally not indicated. Chemotherapy for adenocarcinomas of unknown primary site may fit into this group. These treatments may be rationally allowable if the patient has an adequate reason to justify his desire.

TYPE OF TREATMENT

Standard Treatment

The ability of a particular intervention to accomplish its goal defines the limits of oncology care. When the evidence is strong, and when there are no harms indisputably greater than the harm eliminated, relieved or prevented, the treatment is medically appropriate, and morally permissible if the patient desires it. Highly Indicated and Indicated treatment plans need no justification. Contraindicated and

Non-indicated interventions are not medically acceptable, and must be justified on the rare occasion that a doctor or his patient desires them.

Though in a cost conscious society it would seem wise to put limits on the use of contraindicated and non-indicated cancer treatments, it is sometimes difficult to adhere to such an evidence-based standard.[61]

Innovative Treatment

Where the standard of evidence is weak (Group C) treatments should be regarded as innovative. This designation extends across the spectrum of harms and benefits to include treatments in the following categories: Possibly Beneficial, Equivocal, and Possibly Harmful. It is the doctor's duty to communicate this to his patient whether or not he is a subject in a formal research study under the protection of an Institutional Review Board.

Since most cancer treatments fall into one of these categories, cancer patients are often asked to decide about the desirability of a medical intervention that is not a medically accepted treatment. Therefore, doctors are on higher moral ground when they present these innovative treatments as part of a formal research study. This is, however, not always practicable. "N-of-1" trials,[62] and time-limited trials are alternative approaches.

Deciding to limit access to innovative treatment to patients enrolled on formal studies may be tempting, but this runs the risk of hindering progress and depriving large numbers of cancer patients of Possibly Beneficial Treatments. A more rational approach might be to distinguish between the categories of innovative treatment, and limit access to Equivocal and Possibly Harmful treatments to some form of protocol study.

GOAL OF TREATMENT: CURE VS. PALLIATION

Regardless of whether the treatment is standard or innovative, doctors have a moral duty to provide their patients with comprehensible, adequate information about it, and the alternatives. Oncologists fail in their duty when their patients do not adequately understand whether the goal of treatment is cure or palliation,[63] and, if it is the latter, whether the intent of the palliative treatment is to prolong life or to control symptoms. Truly informed consent requires this information.

Cancer patients routinely overestimate the value of their treatments: be they patients with breast cancer receiving potentially curative adjuvant chemotherapy;[64] patients with metastatic cancer receiving potentially palliative chemotherapy;[65] or patients with refractory cancer receiving chemotherapy as part of phase I clinical trials.[66] Their enthusiasm for chemotherapy is not always shared by others;[67] not even their oncologists.

In a recent survey, the vast majority of Maryland medical oncologists believed strongly in the value of first-line chemotherapy for metastatic breast cancer. They were, however, unenthusiastic about second-line regimens. Despite their attitude, they had little hesitation in recommending second-line treatments for their patients.[68]

The stage is set for arguments over the futility of care when patients and their families develop unrealistic hopes and expectations because their doctors have not adequately discussed the goals of treatment. Without undermining hope, or paternalistically imposing our ranking of the harms and benefits, doctors can, and are duty bound, to advise patients whether a medically acceptable treatment is palliative or curative, and, for example, indicated or possibly harmful.

Oncologists are used to thinking about and accepting goals that are less than absolute. Although we prefer that our treatments produce complete responses, we know that this occurs infrequently, and we have come to count partial responses and even disease stabilization as acceptable and "good." We are often criticized for putting too much emphasis on the rate of response and not its duration. Cure is desirable, but our goals are usually more modest: prolonging life or simply the relief of symptoms. Perhaps oncologists are so used to dealing on the margins of efficacy that they do not experience futility, as a "profound sense of disproportion,"[69] in the same way that other doctors do when they face treatment options with extremely high harm - benefit rations.

Medical oncologists are different. When compared to non-oncologists caring for cancer patients, we tend to write DNR orders much later in the course of our patients' disease. However, our decisions to withhold life-sustaining treatment tend to be more all encompassing than those of our non-oncologist colleagues.[70] Though we tend to fight longer and harder, when it's over it's over. This is reflected in our use of hospice and our efforts to provide quality comfort care at the end of life. Patients with cancer are more likely to opt for intensive chemotherapy than people who do not have cancer. Similarly, medical oncologists' are more likely to accept aggressive treatments for potentially small benefits than non-medical oncologists.[68]

NEXT STEPS

There is certainly no rational reason to continue the practice of blindly administering chemotherapy without defined end points and time lines. Oncologists must prospectively define realistic goals for the treatment that their patients are to receive, and, with their patients, they must monitor the balance of harms. The vast majority of these goals will be measurable end points (a tumor getting smaller, or a symptom relieved), but some, like those of the Russian immigrant waiting to see has daughter, may be more symbolic.

Established early in the course of cancer treatment, expectations and alternatives can be built into "next step" scenarios for our patients and their families. This preventive ethics approach was used successfully to diffuse the inevitable arguments about the futility of ventilator support in the Russian patient with advanced pancreatic cancer. The circumstances of most cancer patients are well suited to similarly designed action plans and decision trees. These "next steps" are as likely to be plans for second line chemotherapy as they are for hospice care. As doctors and patients share their goals and values, rational limits can usually be placed on cancer care.

REFERENCES

1. In the Matter of Karen Ann Quinlan, an alleged incompetent. 355A. 2d 647; or 70 NJ 10. March 31, 1976.

2. In Re: The Conservatorship of Helga M. Wanglie, PX-91-283, Fourth Judicial District (District Court Probate Court Div.) Hennepin County, Minnesota.

3. In the Matter of Baby K, 16 F.3d 590 (4th Cir. 1994).

4. Paris JJ, Crone RK, Reardon F. Physicians' refusal of requested treatment: The case of Baby L. N Engl J Med. 1990;322:1012-1015.

5. Kolta G. Court ruling limits rights of patients: care deemed futile may be withheld. New York Times. 1995 April 22; Sect A-6.

6. Roberts D. Wife battles Winnipeg hospital to keep husband alive. Toronto Globe and Mail. 1998 Nov 10; Sect A-3.

7. Crippen D. Dealing with families who demand inappropriate medical treatment for moribund patients. Intensive Care World. 1992;9:78-80.

8. Lo B, Jonsen AR. Ethical decisions in the care of a patient terminally ill with metastatic cancer. Ann Int Med. 1980;92:107-111.

9. Heffner JE, Brow LK, Barbieri CA. Publications in subspecialty journals on end-of-life ethics. Arch Int Med. 1991;157:685-690.

10. Blackhall LJ. Must we always use CPR? N Engl J Med. *1987;317:1281-1285.*

11. Tomlinson T, Brody H. Ethics and communication in do-not-resuscitate orders. N Engl J Med. 1988;318:43-46.

12. Lantos JD, Singer PA, Walker RM, Gramelspacher GP, Shapiro GR, Sanchez-Gonzalez MA, Stocking CB, Miles SH, Siegler M. The illusion of futility in clinical practice. Am J Med. 1989;87:81-84.

13. Shapiro GR. Unpublished Medline keyword search. Oct. 1998.

14. Bailer JC 3rd, Gornik HL. Cancer undefeated. N Engl J Med. 1997;336:1569-1574.

15. Faber-Lagendoen, K. Resuscitation of patients with metastatic cancer. Arch Int Med. 1991;151:235-239.

16. Kitzhaber JA. The Oregon health plan: a process for reform. Ann Emergency Med. 1994;23:330-333.

17. Jeker NS, Schneidermann LJ. When families request that everything possible be done. J Med & Philosophy. 1995;20:145-163.

18. Escalante CP, Martin CG, Elting LS, et al. Dyspnea in cancer patients: etiology, resource utilization and survival - implications in a managed care world. Cancer. 1996;78:1320-1325.

19. Rubenfeld GD, Crawford SW. Withdrawing life support from mechanically ventilated recipients of bone marrow transplants: a case for evidence-based guidelines. Ann Int Med. 1996;125:625-633.

20. American Medical Association Council on Ethical and Judicial Affairs. Medical futility in end-of-life care. JAMA. 1999;281:937-941.

21. American Thoracic Society Bioethics Task Force. Withholding and withdrawing life-sustaining therapy. Am Rev Respir Dis. 1991;144:726-731.

22. Bedell SE, Delbanco TL, Cook EF, Epstein FH. Survival after cardiopulmonary resuscitation in the hospital. N Engl J Med. 1983;309:569-576.

23. Schneiderman LJ, Jecker NS, Jonsen AR. Medical futility: its meaning and ethical implications. Ann Intern Med. 1990;112:949-954.

24. Schneiderman LJ, Faber-Langendoen K, Jecker NS. Am J Med. 1994;96:110-114.

25. Truog RD, Brett AS, Frader J. The problem with futility. N Engl J Med. 1992;326:1560-1564.

26. Vitelli CE, Cooper K, Rogatko A, Brennan MF. Cardiopulmonary resuscitation and the patient with cancer. J Clin Oncol. 1991;9:111-115.

27. Truog RD. Progress in the futility debate. J Clinical Ethics. 1995;6:128-132.

28. Solomon MZ. How physicians talk about futility: making word mean too many things. J of Law Med & Ethics. 1993;21:231-237.

29. Curtis RJ, Park DR, Krone MR, Pearlman RA. Use of the medical futility rationale in do-not-attempt-resuscitation orders. JAMA. 1995;273:124-128.

30. Zawacki BE. The "futility debate" and the management of Gordian knots. J Clinical Ethics. 1995;6:112-127.

31. Katz J. *The Silent World of Doctor and Patient.* New York: Free Press. 1997.

32. American College of Physicians Ethics Manual. Ann Intern Med. 1998;128:576-594.

33 Caralis PV, Davis B, Wright K, Marcial E. The influence of ethnicity and race on attitudes toward advance directives, life-prolonging treatments, and euthanasia. J Clinical Ethics. 1993;4:155-165.

34 United States Department of Health and Human Services Policy for the Protection of Human Subjects. Fed Register. Vol 46, No 17:8951. January 27, 1981.

35 President's Commission for the Study of Ethical Problems in Medicine and Biomedical and Behavioral Research. *Making Health Care Decisions: the Ethical and Legal Implications of Informed Consent in the Patient-Practitioner Relationship.* Washington, DC: Government Printing Office. 1982:42-44.

36. Gert B, Culver CM, Clouser KD. *Bioethics: a return to fundamentals.* New York: Oxford University Press. 1997:93-130.

37. Gert B. *Morality: a new justification of the Moral rules.* New York: Oxford University Press. 1988.

38. Brett AS, McCulloug LB. When patients request specific interventions: defining the limits of the physician's obligation. N Engl J Med. 1986;315:1347-1351.

39. President's Commission for the Study of Ethical Problems in Medicine and Biomedical and Behavioral Research. *Deciding to Forego Life-Sustaining Treatment.* Washington, DC: Government Printing Office. 1983.

40. Wanzer SH, Adelstein SJ, Cranford RE, et al. The physician's responsibility toward hopelessly ill patients. N Engl J Med. 1984;310:955-959.

41. Shapiro GR. Not telling Russian immigrants the truth about cancer: cultural sensitivity or misplaced paternalism? Psycho-oncology. 1996;5:196.

42. Gert B, Culver CM, Clouser KD. 1997:149-180.

43. Brock DW, Wartman SA. When competent patients make irrational choices. N Engl J Med. 1990;322:1595-1599.

44. Gert B. 1988: 286-295.

45. Gert B, Culver CM, Clouser KD. 1997:26-31.

46. Doukas DJ, McCullough LB. A preventive ethics approach to counseling patients about clinical futility in the primary care setting. Arch Fam Med. 1996;5:589-592.

47. Solomon MZ, O'Donnell L, Jennings B, et al. Decisions near the end of life: professional views on life-sustaining treatments. Am J Public Health. 1993;83:14-23.

48. Jecker NS, Schneiderman LJ. Futility and rationing. Am J Med. 1992;92:189-196.

49. Studnicki J, Schapira DV, Straumfjord JV, et al. A national profile of the use of intensive care by Medicare patients with cancer. Cancer. 1994;74:2366-2373.

50. Gatter RA, Moskop JC. From futility to triage. J of Med and Philos. 1995;20:191-205.

51. DeLima M, Ghaddar H, Pierce S, Estey E. Treatment of newly-diagnosed acute myelogenous leukaemia in patients aged 80 years and above. Br J Haematology. 1996;93:89-95.

52. Kitagawa T, Hara M, Sano T, Sugimura T. The concept of tenju-gann, or "natural-end cancer." Cancer. 1998;83:1061-5.

53. Callahan D. *What Kind of Life: The limits of medical progress.* New York: Simon & Schuster. 1990.

54. Slevin ML. Quality of life: philosophical questions or clinical reality? Br Med J. 1992;305:466-469.

55. O'Connor AMC, Boyd NF, Padraig W, Stolbach L, Till JE. Eliciting preferences for alternative drug therapies in oncology: influence of treatment outcome description, elicitation technique and treatment experience on preferences. J Chron Dis. 1987;40:811-818.

56. Tsevat J, Dawson NV, Wu AW, et al. Health values of Hospitalized patients 80 years or older. JAMA. 1998;279:371-375.

57. Hamel MB, Teno JM, Goldman L, et al. Patient age and decisions to withhold life-sustaining treatments from seriously ill, hospitalized adults. Ann Intern Med. 1999;130:116-125.

58. Cassileth BR, Zupkis RV, Sutton-Smith K, March BA. Information and participation preferences among cancer patients. Ann Intern Med. 1980;92:832-836.

59. U.S. Preventive Services Task Force. *Guide to Clinical Preventive Services: An Assessment of the Effectiveness of 169 Interventions.* Baltimore: Williams & Wilkins. 1989.

60. Sharpe VA, Faden AI. Appropriateness in patient care: a new conceptual framework. Milbank Quarterly. 1996;74:115-138.

61. Rosenbaum S, Frankford DM, Moor B, Borzi P. Who should determine when health care is medically necessary? N Engl J Med. 1999;340:229-232.

62. Guyatt GH, Keller JL, Jaeschke R, et al. The n-of-1 randomized controlled trial: clinical usefulness. Our three-year experience. Ann Intern Med. 1990;112:293-299.

63. Gregory DR, Cotler MP. Futility: are goals the problem? Part two. Cambridge Quarterly of Healthcare Ethics. 1994;3:125-134.

64. Ravdin PM, Siminoff IA, Harvey JA. Survey of breast cancer patients concerning their knowledge and expectations of adjuvant therapy. J Clin Oncol. 1998;16:515-521.

65. Weeks JC, Cook EF, O'Day SJ, et al. Relationship between cancer patients' predictions of prognosis and their treatment preferences. JAMA. 1998;279:1709-1714.

66. Daugherty C, Ratain MJ, Grochowski E, et al. Perceptions of cancer patients and their physicians involved in phase I trials. J Clin Oncol. 1995;13:1062-1072.

67. Slevin ML, Stubbs L, Plant H, et al. Attitudes to chemotherapy: comparing views of patients with those of doctors, nurses, and general public. Br Med J. 1990;300:1458-1460.

68. Benner SE, Fetting JH, Brenner MH. A stopping rule for standard chemotherapy for metastatic breast cancer: lessons from a survey of Maryland medical oncologists. Cancer Investigation. 1994;12:451-455.

69. Prendergast TJ. Futility and the common cold: how requests for antibiotics can illuminate care at the end of life. Chest. 1995;107:836-844.

70. Shapiro GR, Stocking CB, LaPuma J, Silverstein MD, Roland D, Siegler M. Do not resuscitate orders & life-sustaining therapy: a comparison of oncologists' & nononcologists' attitudes. Proc Am Soc Clin Oncol. 1988;7:269.

6 ROLE OF PALLIATIVE MEDICINE IN CANCER PATIENT CARE

Charles F. von Gunten, M.D., Ph.D.
Jeanne Martinez, R.N., M.P.H.

INTRODUCTION

There continues to be an unexplained paradox in American cancer care. On the one hand, of all Americans who have cancer, only 50% will be cured.[1,2] Most of these cures are due to surgical intervention. This proportion has remained relatively unchanged over the past 30 years. During the course of their illness for those patients whose cancer is not cured, most patients will experience considerable suffering. That suffering has physical, psychological (emotional), social (practical) and spiritual components. Multiple studies have demonstrated that these elements of patients' and families' suffering are not met by the current medical system.[3,4,5]

On the other hand, academic oncology has resisted addressing this issue of broad importance and applicability. Medical School and residency curricula have devoted little, if any time, to the subject. Only a handful of faculty are supported to develop expertise in this area. Most of the cancer centers supported by the National Cancer Institute do not have clinical programs or research programs aimed at reducing the suffering of this large number of patients.

It is the purpose of this chapter to define the role of palliative medicine in cancer care. First, palliative medicine will be defined. Then, a conceptual framework for its role in the comprehensive care of patients with cancer will be presented. Finally, an example of how clinical palliative care may be integrated into a cancer center will be described.

PALLIATIVE MEDICINE

Since the time of Hippocrates there have been two overall goals of medical care:

1) Cure of Disease
2) Relief of Suffering

The relative emphasis on cure versus relief of suffering relates to both the underlying medical condition and the overall goals of the person who has the illness.

Palliative Medicine is the term coined to denote the field of medicine concerned with the relief of suffering and the improvement of quality of life. Quality-of-life rather than quantity-of-life is the chief aim of those engaged in the delivery of palliative care.[6]   Because suffering is experienced by persons, its existence, character and criteria for relief is defined by the patient rather than by the physician. Because persons do not exist in isolation, the relief of suffering requires attention to the care of patients and their families. Suffering is caused by many factors that are rarely limited to the physical domain. In providing whole person care to relieve suffering, palliative medicine attends to all domains of the human experience of illness that may be involved: physical, psychological, social and spiritual.[7,8] Tending to the relief of suffering in these domains cannot possibly be accomplished by a single medical discipline – a team approach is required. Therefore, palliative medicine may be defined in the following way:

> *Palliative Medicine: the interdisciplinary care of patients focussing on the relief of suffering and the improvement of quality of life.*

The Royal College of Physicians in Great Britain recognized palliative medicine as a physician specialty in 1987.[9] This recognition came only after it had been demonstrated that there was an established body of medical knowledge that uniquely pertained to a distinct patient population. Further, there was recognition of a 4-year training program to follow general medical training for those physicians wishing to be recognized as specialists in the field. Subsequently, the Royal College of Physicians and Surgeons in Australia recognized the specialty. The Royal College of Physicians and Surgeons and the College of Family Practice of Canada will soon make a similar move (L.Librach, personal communication).

Progress towards this goal in the US has been hindered by the fact that hospice programs were introduced and established in the United States in a manner different from that in other countries. Nurses or volunteers established the majority of programs as a reaction against the perceived inadequacies of the medical establishment in caring for terminally ill patients. Until recently, physician participation has not been prominent. Consequently, there developed a polarity that prevented hospice medicine from becoming incorporated into the academic mainstream. Despite this separation from mainstream medicine, the hospice movement in the United States has grown to include more than 2500 individual hospice programs caring for about 1/3 of the US population who die of cancer each year.[10]

Fortunately, there are initiatives in a few of the cancer centers in the United States that suggest that mainstream medicine and palliative care are negotiating a rapprochement. Nearly every national organization is calling for increased clinical and academic focus in Hospice and Palliative Medicine including the Institute of Medicine,[11] the National Institutes of Health,[12] the American Board of Internal Medicine,[13] the American College of Physicians,[14] the American Society of Oncology,[15] and the American Medical Association.[16] In particular, the Institute of Medicine has called for a cadre of physicians with special expertise in this area to enable patient care, education, and research.[11]

Conceptual Framework

The concepts that undergird the field of Palliative Medicine have only been articulated in the past century and have arisen in reaction to the single-minded application of the scientific method in medicine. The relief of suffering as a goal of medical care was subjugated or lost in many settings in the quest to achieve cure and/or prolongation of life. While the impetus for the rigor of science to provide insight into cancer and its treatment is unquestionable, it should not obliterate the emphasis on caring for the human being who has the disease. It is a mistaken assertion that treating the cancer is equivalent to treating a person with cancer. This model has led contemporary oncology to cause suffering in some circumstances. The distinction between disease and illness is critical for chronic progressive cancer that is incurable. The misapplication of an exclusively "cure-oriented" approach to cancer can be conceptualized in the following diagram where the time course and goals of such treatment are illustrated (Figure 1).

Figure 1: Curative/Life-Prolonging Therapy

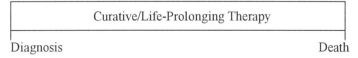

A patient is first evaluated for some constellation of symptoms for which a diagnosis of cancer is made. Evaluation and treatment is directed toward the eradication, reversal, or substantial control of the disease. Symptoms are important insofar as they help elucidate the diagnosis and course of treatment. This model of treatment can be characterized as disease-oriented and pathophysiologically based. Clinicians are engaged in a "war on cancer" and the patient dies in spite of "doing everything" and maintaining a "fighting spirit" to the end.

It should be apparent that this model may actually cause suffering. It also promotes the ethically dubious practice of administering anti-cancer therapy that will have no benefit, but may be perceived as still trying to "fight" the cancer. It is this orientation, however well-meaning, that has led to the disparaging way that clinicians outside of medical oncology refer to medical oncologists. There is that gruesome joke that still makes the rounds, "Why do they put nails in coffins? To keep the oncologists out".

In recognition of the situation when the disease is progressive and treatment modalities are no longer effective, "comfort care" measures may be instituted. This last period, if it occurs at all, is often of short duration (sometimes hours to days). Furthermore, this medical care model does not include explicit consideration of non-physical aspects of a person's illness experience or that of the person's family. This model of medical care leads to several important sources of societal dissatisfaction with the medical field—physicians "over-treat", physicians "don't give patients enough information about their condition and what to expect", and physicians are "merely scientists who are uninterested in the lives of the patients they treat". Further, once "comfort care" has been recommended, there is an accurate perception that the physicians are often no longer engaged in the care of the patient. Physicians, in their defense, will say that their job is to treat the cancer. When they can't treat the cancer anymore, there is nothing for them to do. This orientation misses some of the fundamental ethical imperatives of the profession.

For physicians who try to modify the approach diagrammed in figure 1 to include only medical care which is appropriate for the stage of disease and the likely outcomes of treatment, the patient and family may perceive the care to be more like that shown in Figure 2:

Figure 2: Curative/Life-Prolonging Therapy with Comfort Care

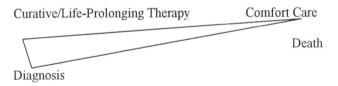

Curative/Life-Prolonging Therapy   Comfort Care

                                          Death

Diagnosis

The patient and family perceive, often quite correctly, that the physician shows diminished attention to the patient over time. This leads to another fundamental cause for patient and family dissatisfaction with the health care system--abandonment. Although the severity of illness may be increasing, the attention of the physician and other health care providers diminishes when there is "nothing more to do" for the disease. In addition, the implication of abandonment may lead to strident demands from patients and families to "do more, do everything". In the absence of an appropriate treatment framework that addresses these issues, the physician may pursue medical treatment that is futile in the service of patient autonomy. Such treatment results in more suffering for the patient and family because the important issues that surround death and dying are ignored.

In appreciation that the models diagrammed in Figures 1 and 2 do not adequately address issues of patient suffering, Dr. Cicely Saunders in England introduced the hospice model of palliative care.[8] Working primarily with patients with cancer, she recognized that suffering might be produced not only from the cancer, but also by medical efforts to control the disease. She also recognized that the physical, psychological, social, and spiritual aspects of suffering were inadequately addressed. Culminating in the establishment of St. Christopher's Hospice in south suburban London in 1967, she developed a model of inpatient care for patients for whom curative therapy was not available, or was no longer desired. In this model there is an interdisciplinary team approach to the care of the patient and family that continues into a bereavement period after the patient's death. The hospice concept has been widely adopted because of its demonstrated benefits for patients and families. Figure 3 shows the most common position of hospice care in the overall scheme introduced in Figure 1. There is generally a sharp demarcation between disease-oriented therapy and hospice care.

Figure 3: The Hospice Care Position

Curative/Life-Prolonging Therapy	Hospice Care

Although hospice care addresses aspects of patient suffering not addressed during "standard medical treatment", this period is often short (median of 30 days in the US) and there is a sharp discontinuity between the previous medical care and hospice care. Conceptually, one of the chief problems with this model is the dichotomy between curative/life-prolonging care and hospice care. This model suggests that the goal of medical care is *first* cure, *then* relief of suffering. Yet, good sense dictates that the two goals can be pursued simultaneously. Why wait to introduce measures to alleviate suffering and improve quality of life until all attempts at cure have been exhausted or the patient and family plead for such efforts to stop? It would seem to be generally appropriate to integrate cure/prolongation of life treatment with the relief of suffering. The nature and course of the illness and the patient and family's goals for care should determine the relative emphasis on cure versus palliation. It should be self-evident that many palliative care approaches to illness should precede the point at which referral to a hospice program is appropriate. For example, aggressive control of pain, other bothersome symptoms, and the psychosocial effects of a cancer diagnosis should characterize the very *beginning* of contemporary cancer care. This approach can accompany aggressive anti-cancer therapy with curative or life-prolonging intent (such as in lymphoma or breast cancer) as well as for diseases where death is inevitable. This scheme is shown in Figure 4.

Figure 4: A Better Approach

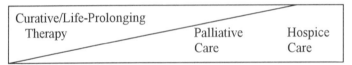

In this model, Hospice Care represents the completion of medical care, not an alternative to, or an abrupt change from, the preceding care plan.[17]

As disease progresses, inpatient hospital treatment has conventionally increased. The number of admissions to inpatient settings and the use of health care resources increases dramatically during the last year of a patient's life. To minimize patient suffering during this period, as well as to ameliorate the contribution that inpatient treatment makes to suffering, hospice programs in the US have pursued the provision of palliative care at home. Most patients find this preferable to institutional care, but not all. Therefore, a program of palliative medicine must coordinate and deliver care across a continuum to encompass all phases of illness and locations of medical treatment in order to care for the patient and family in the best possible way.

PROGRAM OF PALLIATIVE CARE

Many people and institutions have expressed interest in developing programs of hospice and palliative care. There is a paucity of information in the literature about how such programs might be organized and financed.[18] Yet, if the poor quality of palliation practiced in American cancer centers is to be improved, then palliative medicine must be firmly established in the cancer centers that care for Americans. There should not be a false dichotomy between "care" and "cure". Patients must not feel they have to choose between a miserable life or hastened death. The ongoing debate in the US over physician-assisted suicide, including the recent US Supreme Court decision on the subject, will continue to emphasize the need for the provision of palliative care to all citizens.

Northwestern Memorial Hospital (NMH) is the principal teaching affiliate hospital of Northwestern University Medical School. It is a 773-bed private, non-profit hospital located in the urban center of the city of Chicago. It has all departments of a general hospital with the exception of pediatrics. Although the Dean of the medical school sits on its Board of Directors, its governance and financing are separate from the university. In fiscal year 1997, the hospital recorded 36,450 admissions, an increase of 5% over fiscal year 1996. Average length of stay for the hospital as a whole was 4.29 days. There were 698 deaths in the hospital (including the emergency department) in fiscal 1997.

A program of home-based nursing-run supportive care was conceived in 1980 and instituted by the hospital in 1982 in response to the need to develop more community outreach. The hospice appellation was specifically excluded because of the opposition of the attending physician staff at the time. Beginning in 1985, with the initiation of state licensure for hospice, elements of a conventional hospice program were added and it was officially denoted as the Hospice Program of Northwestern Memorial Hospital by 1986. Medical Direction and its connection to the medical school were formalized in the Division of Hematology/Oncology, Department of Medicine.

In 1987 a 10-bed inpatient unit on an existing hospital ward was opened in response to a philanthropic gift for the renovation and establishment of such an inpatient unit. Although the costs of renovation of the unit were enabled by philanthropy, fee-for-service billing provided operating revenues. In 1993 a consultation service which operated in the rest of the hospital was instituted. In 1997 the name of the program was changed to the Palliative Care and Home Hospice Program in recognition of the increased scope of activities and patients for whom the program was able to care. In this regard, it is interesting to note that the program specifically resisted becoming certified for the Medicare Hospice Benefit until 1991 because of the risk that good palliative care would be defined by the restrictions of a reimbursement mechanism rather than by principles of palliative medicine. However, in response to evidence that appropriate patients were not able to be served without such certification, application was made and accepted. However, on a national basis, one of the most significant barriers to the integration of hospice care into the mainstream of medicine has been the tendency to define appropriate patient care by the regulations pertaining to the Hospice Medicare Benefit reimbursement mechanism.

The Strategic Plan of the Northwestern Memorial Corporation for its integrated health care system (of which NMH is a part) articulates the vision for the entire medical center in terms of a transition from a traditional inpatient hospital to a local, integrated health care delivery system that provides care across a continuum of patient care needs. In an analogous way, the Palliative Care and Home Hospice Program is developing in such a way as to bridge the continuum of palliative care needs for patients and families. The program strives to no longer be "an alternative" to other types of medical care; rather, to be the completion of good medical care. In many ways, the program exemplifies many aspects of the aspirations of the medical center as a whole--appropriate, quality care that is delivered in the setting that is best for the patient and family.

The delivery of health care services for patients with cancer can be conceptualized as a continuum from acute hospital settings, to skilled and custodial nursing facilities, to ambulatory care facilities, to the patient's own home. The Palliative Care and Home Hospice Program currently conducts patient care in three different areas in the spectrum of health care. In the acute general hospital it provides recommendations and assistance through its Hospice/Palliative Medicine Consultation Service. There is an inpatient unit for the acute palliative care of patients who are too ill to be cared for in other settings. Finally, the program provides home hospice services either as a sole agency or in cooperation with Northwestern Home Health Care—a home healthcare agency. Patients in the home hospice program may be admitted to the inpatient unit, if needed. Patients may also be seen in the ambulatory outpatient oncology office.   A summary of the characteristics of each of these current areas of service follows.

Components of the Northwestern Program

Consultation Service

The consultation service and the nature of the palliative medicine consultation have been described elsewhere in detail.[19]   A nurse, an attending physician, and rotating fellows, housestaff, and medical students staff the service.   Patients are seen anywhere in the hospital at the request of the managing service. During fiscal year 1997, an average of 57 consultations (range 45-80) was requested each month. This average has increased approximately 5% per year since the inception of the service in 1993.   The service is widely perceived as helpful by medical center physicians and staff.

Acute Inpatient Palliative Care Unit

The inpatient unit has been described elsewhere in detail.[20,21]   It currently consists of 12 acute hospital beds in large private rooms on a dedicated nursing unit in the hospital.   The average inpatient census at midnight for fiscal year 1996 was 9.5. The midnight census is the count of patients who are alive at midnight occupying a bed on the unit.   Patients who were admitted and died before midnight, discharged home before midnight, or admitted after midnight are not counted as part of the daily census.   Consequently, there have been as many as 16 different patients who come through the unit in a given 24 hour period even though the midnight census indicates only 8 patients on that day.   Although this convention for measuring occupancy underrates the overall workload of the unit, this is the convention that is widely used in the hospital industry for reporting and billing for occupancy. A 43% increase in average census in 1994 is related to the institution of the consultation service.   In fact, the number of beds on the inpatient unit was increased from 10 to 12 in 1995 in order to accommodate the increase in demand. There was a drop in average census in 1997 to 6.5 related to the introduction of protease inhibitors in the treatment of AIDS.   In 1994 almost 25% of patients had AIDS as their primary diagnosis.   In 1997 only 7% of patients had AIDS. The average midnight census has increased to 9 in the third quarter of fiscal year 1998.

Of the 459 patients hospitalized on the unit in fiscal year 1996, 54 % had Medicare, 13% had Medicaid (or Medicaid-pending) and 33% had commercial insurance.   Of those with commercial insurance, less than 10% were in an HMO. Virtually all of the remainder represented PPO indemnity plans.   Only 2 patients were uninsured.   This breakdown is essentially the same as for patients seen by the consultation service. The unit has a distinctive design to accommodate families in a more home-like atmosphere.   Visiting hours, ages and numbers of visitors are unrestricted. Pets may visit and patients may smoke cigarettes. The unit is staffed with full-time professional staff and hospice-trained volunteers. Some professional staff and volunteers are shared with the home hospice program. For example, the bereavement coordinator works to extend bereavement support to all families of those who die either on the unit or at home. Because it is an acute care unit, the full range of services and treatments available in an acute hospital are available. The only requirements for admission are a "do-not-resuscitate" order and a primarily palliative focus of medical treatment. Direct admission from home or office without being evaluated in the emergency department is permitted at all hours. Enrollment in a home hospice program is not required.

There is a high degree of patient, family, and physician satisfaction as measured by survey data. In annual surveys, patients and family rank the quality of care as among the highest in the hospital. Similarly, surveys of attending staff rank the quality of the nursing as among the highest in the institution.

All insurers and third party payers that cover hospitalization at NMH cover hospitalization on the unit. Patients are not required to have accessed hospice insurance benefits to be admitted. Appropriateness of admission and continued stay are evaluated using the same criteria for utilization review as other patients in the hospital.[22] Despite changes in guidelines for overall utilization, the denial rate for inpatient charges remains among the lowest in the hospital. However, the utilization review department is actively engaged in negotiating and defending the admission of patients to the unit. Many cases go on to review and appeal before they are ultimately paid.

Home Hospice Program

Medicare and the Joint Commission on Accreditation of Healthcare Organizations certify the home hospice program. The team delivers hospice care to patients and families living within the city limits of Chicago. The average census fluctuates between 35 and 50 patients per day. In fiscal year 1997 the program cared for 198 patients at home. The median length of stay is 31 days with an average of 73.9 days. The median length of stay increased from an average of 19 days in 1993 after the introduction of the consultation service. In contrast with the inpatient and consultation services, the payer source for 125 patients cared for at home in fiscal year 1997 was 68% Medicare, 15% public aid, and 10% commercial payer. Six percent of patients at home were uninsured. The program uses the NMH indigent care budget to provide basic hospice care at home that would conform to that provided by the Hospice Medicare Benefit without regard to financial situation. Further, the program uses philanthropy to provide care that would not otherwise be available – principally the hiring of caregivers for patients who live alone or who have frail or working caregivers. We do not use philanthropy for the basic hospice care that would be covered by the NMH indigent budget.

As with other home hospice programs, the program prevents unnecessary admissions to acute hospital and skilled nursing facilities and avoids unnecessary use of the emergency department by having nurses on-call 24 hours per day, 7 days per week to provide a rapid response to changes in symptoms. The program works flexibly to coordinate care with Northwestern Home Health Agency, a separate home health agency owned by the hospital corporation to maximize patient benefit.

Program Summary

The program has had a marked effect on the location of death for patients in the hospital. The total number of deaths in the hospital (including those in the emergency department) has remained remarkably constant at approximately 700 patients per year since 1990 despite an increase in admissions of approximately 6% per year. Over the period from 1990 to 1997 the percent of people dying in the intensive care units, operating rooms, and emergency department has remained approximately 40%. However, the number of patients dying in the inpatient palliative care unit has increased from 25% to 38% (22). This has been accompanied by a concomitant decrease in deaths on the general medical and surgical units. Given the better attention to palliative care on a dedicated unit, and the more appropriate utilization of health care resources that occur there, this is a large effect on the care of the dying in the hospital.

Despite being a teaching hospital, NMH is a private hospital where the medical staff is composed of approximately half full-time faculty and half private-practitioners. Patients are admitted to the hospital, and admitted to the home hospice program, under the patient's primary attending. More than half of the 219 physicians who admitted patients to the unit were general internists (there are no family physicians on staff at the hospital). Only 14% of the physicians were oncologists despite more than half of patients having a diagnosis of cancer. Nine percent of the attendings were surgeons. This is evidence of the broad acceptance and integration of the program into the culture of the medical center.[23]

CONCLUSION

Until we can reliably, predictably, and easily cure cancer, it is imperative that the principles of palliative care be incorporated into mainstream comprehensive cancer programs. Hospice care, and the aspects of palliative care that are pertinent throughout the course of the illness, should be a part of every program. This has been recognized by the Commission on Cancer in its new certification guidelines and advocated by the American Society of Clinical Oncology. A program that includes consultation, inpatient, and home components is required.

REFERENCES

1. Bailar JC III, Gornick HC. Cancer undefeated. N Engl J Med 1997;336:1569-74.

2. Bailar JC III, Smtih EM. Progress against cancer? N Engl J Med 1986;314:1226-32.

3. The SUPPORT Principal Investigators. A controlled trial to improve care for seriously ill hospitalized patients. JAMA 1995;274:1591-1598.

4. Vachon ML, Kristjanson L, Higginson I. Psychosocial issues in palliative care. J Pain Symptom Manage 1995;10:142-50.

5. Vachon ML. Caring for the caregiver in oncology and palliative care. Semin Oncol Nurs 1998;14:152-70.

6. Doyle, D, Hanks GWC, MacDonald N. Introduction. In: *Oxford Textbook of Palliative Medicine*, 2nd edition. Eds: Derek Doyle, Geoffrey W.C. Hanks, Neil MacDonald. Oxford University Press, New York 1998.

7. Cassel EJ. *The nature of suffering and the goals of medicine.* Oxford University Press, New York, 1991.

8. Saunders C. Introduction-History and Challenge. In: *The Management of Terminal Malignant disease.* Eds: Cicely Saunders and Nigel Sykes. Edward Arnold Boston 1993.

9. Doyle D. Palliative medicine: a UK specialty. J Palliat Care 1994;10:8-9.

10. National Hospice Organization. 1901 N. Moore Street, Suite 901 Arlington, VA 22209.

11. Approaching death: improving care at the end of life. Committee on care at the end of life, Division of Health Care Services, Institute of Medicine, national Academy of Sciences, 1997.

12. National Institute of Nursing Research. National Institutes of Health 6701 Rockledge Drive Room 1040 MSC 7710 Bethesda, MD 20892-7710.

13. American Board of Internal Medicine. *Caring for the Dying: identification and promotion of physician competency.* Philadelphia 1996.

14. Cassel C. Palliative care is the real focus of end-of-life medicine. ACP Observer. 1996;July/August:2.

15. Task Force on Cancer Care at the End of Life. Cancer care during the last phase of life. Journal of Clinical Oncology1998;1986-1996.

16. Good care of the dying patient. Council on Scientific Affairs. JAMA 1996;275:474-8.

17. Donald N. The interface between oncology and palliative medicine. In: *Oxford Textbook of Palliative Medicine*, 2nd edition. Eds: Derek Doyle, Geoffrey W.C. Hanks, Neil MacDonald. Oxford University Press, New York 1998.

18. Goldstein P, Walsh D, Horvitz LU. The Cleveland Clinic Foundation Harry R. Horvitz Palliative Care Center. Support Care Cancer 1996;4:329-33.

19. von Gunten CF, Camden B, Neely KJ, Franz G, Martinez J. Prospective evaluation of referrals to a hospice/palliative medicine consultation service. Journal of Palliative Medicine 1998;1(1):45-53.

20. Kellar N, Martinez J, Finis N, Bolger A, von Gunten CF. Characterization of an acute inpatient Hospice Palliative Care Unit in a US teaching hospital. Journal of Nursing Administration 1996;26:16-20.

21. Ng K and von Gunten C. Symptoms and attitudes of 100 consecutive patients admitted to an acute hospice/palliative care unit. Journal of Pain and Symptom Management (in press).

22. von Gunten CF, Martinez J. A program of hospice and palliative care in a private, non-profit US teaching hospital. Journal of Palliative Medicine 1998;1(3)(in press).

23. von Gunten CF, Von Roenn JH, Neely KJ, Martinez J, Weitzman S.   Hospice and palliative care: evaluation of the attitudes and practices of the physician faculty of an academic hospital.   American Journal of Hospice & Palliative Care. 1995;12(4):38-42.

7 INFORMED CONSENT, THE CANCER PATIENT, AND PHASE I CLINICAL TRIALS

Christopher K. Daugherty, M.D.

INTRODUCTION

The concept of informed consent, which acknowledges the rights of patients to voluntarily participate in health care, applies both to clinical practice and clinical research.[1,2] Informed consent in clinical research is related to, but recognized as being more stringent than, informed consent outside the context of clinical trials.[3] This heightened consent standard exists for at least two reasons. First, from an ethical perspective, a patient considering clinical trial participation is always viewed as potentially vulnerable.[4] As a result of this potential vulnerability, he or she may have great difficulty in appreciating the differences between the therapeutic and research aspects of a given alternative of care or treatment. Without this distinction, patients cannot make uncoerced and autonomous health care decisions. Thus, the informed consent process, and the ethics of clinical research, require that such a clear distinction be made.[5,6] Second, the physician-investigator is seen as having an intrinsic conflict of interest in their role both as a physician for an individual patient and as a scientific investigator attempting to develop improved methods of medical care and treatment.[3,4,7] Within the sole context of a therapeutic relationship, the physician places his or her patient's interests above all else.[8] However, within the context of clinical research, an investigator has additional interests which may not be relative to their patients' interests.[9,10,11,12,13] From an ethical perspective, many concerns exist about the ability of clinical investigators to provide the requisite information to patients regarding participation in research in such a way that allows patients to recognize the distinction between research and therapy.[6,14,15]

In an attempt to emphasize the importance of this distinction, most ethical regulations governing clinical research have focused on the informed consent process as a means of protecting potentially vulnerable research subjects from physical and psychological harm.[3,4,16]   These regulations have relied heavily on written informed consent documents to achieve full disclosure of the important elements of consent, including the risks of research participation, the nature of the research, and alternatives to research participation. However, from their inception to the present day, many critics have recognized the imperfect nature of the methods used to regulate the informed consent process.[15,17,18,19,20,21,22] More recent empirical research on informed consent, a great proportion of which as been conducted in the cancer setting, has been very useful in attempting to objectively identify the current problems and deficiencies associated with written consent documents and their oversight.[23,24,25] Over the last 20 years, several of these studies have increasingly demonstrated that although regulations are being followed, informed consent documents have become increasingly unreadable, lengthy, and uninformative. Indeed, they may actually be interfering with what might otherwise be an ethically appropriate informed consent process for patients, including not only those with cancer but any patient considering therapeutic clinical trial participation.

Informed Consent: A Definition and Brief History

A definition of informed consent for clinical research that encompasses all relevant aspects of the process remains somewhat elusive, with varying definitions having been described.[1,2,3,4] Generally, it is viewed as a process of communication between a patient-subject and a clinician-investigator regarding an investigational or experimental treatment. Within this communication process, several elements must be disclosed. These include the disclosure of the type of research to be performed, the risks and benefits of the treatment or research, the unproved nature of the research, the alternatives other than participation in the clinical trial, and finally, disclosure of the subject's freedom to withdraw or not to participate in the research without any detrimental effect on the patient's continued access to adequate health care. Separate from the issue of disclosure within this process is the issue of actual understanding on the part of the patient with regard to these disclosed elements. Whether the definition of informed consent should include an actual understanding of these elements, or how much of an understanding it should include, remain matters of controversy.[1,15,26] However, from an ethical standpoint it is accepted that the process of informed consent requires at least some attempt on the part of the clinician-investigator to help a patient understand those aspects of the consent process which have been disclosed so that the patient may autonomously and voluntarily decide to participate.[27,28] Other elements which have been described as an important part of the informed consent process include maintaining the confidentiality of a research subject's participation and, controversially, possible disclosure of potential conflicts of interest on the part of the clinician-investigator.

This early history of the concept of informed consent appears to relate predominately to patients simply consenting to receive therapy, it does not necessarily relate to disclosure to the patient of the commonly recognized modern day elements of informed consent, e.g., the risks and alternatives of the therapy, let alone an understanding of these elements.[1,2] Regarding informed consent in the therapeutic research setting, evidence of investigators pursuing consent through any concerted and conscientious efforts dates back to only the past fifty years.[1,2,29,30] Although there is some historical evidence that earlier clinical researchers were sensitive to the importance of subjects' consent to research,[31] this appears to have been relevant only from the standpoint that it was viewed as freeing the experimenter from culpability in the event of harm coming to the subject. As well, it is informed consent within the research setting of the last half century that has employed some of the more recent concepts, including use of a written consent document and seeking actual understanding on the part of the research subject, rather than simple disclosure, of the elements of consent.

Informed consent, either as a concept or the term itself, has quite commonly (and perhaps mistakenly) been traced to the Nuremberg Code.[1,14] Yet, as a code written in response to crimes against humanity, and more specifically written with regard to non-therapeutic human subject research, the Nuremberg Code had little impact on the actual practice of therapeutic clinical research at the time of its writing. As well, the code did not specifically mention informed consent. In fact, the term informed consent was believed by many to have first been used in a 1957 malpractice case, Salgo versus Leland Stanford Jr. University.[32,33,34] In this case, the California Supreme Court stated that no patient can submit to a medical intervention without having given prior "informed consent". This ruling has been referenced for more than 45 years by medical historians, legal analysts and medical ethicists as the event from which the term first originated.

More recently, however, the final report of the President's Advisory Committee on Human Radiation Experiments (ACHRE) provides an earlier, and perhaps more interesting, history with regard to the term "informed consent".[35] Through the committee's extensive research of archival materials from the Atomic Energy Commission (AEC), a little known letter was rediscovered, written in 1947 to a clinical investigator from the general manager of the newly formed AEC on an obscure and new requirement regarding the need for "informed consent". The letter was written specifically in response to the investigator's request to allow the declassification of data from government-sponsored radiation research on cancer patients, in order that it might be reported and published by the investigator. As exemplified in the letter, the newly formed AEC clearly had significant concerns over potential litigation and public perception problems regarding the use of seemingly vulnerable cancer patients as subjects of research without any documentation of consent. It will undoubtedly require further examination of these historical foundations of informed consent to know what impact these early and vague policies had on subsequent guidelines and regulations developed by the U.S. Federal Government in the regulatory conduct of clinical research. Yet, there is some evidence to suggest that these early policies did influence the subsequent guidelines developed and used in establishing the National Institute of Health Clinical Center (NIH), and in Government-sponsored research within the Department of Defense and branches of the armed services.[36] Whatever the case, this history clearly shows that informed consent, either as a term or a concept, was discussed within the context of clinical research a full decade prior to its previously recognized origins within the realm of medical malpractice and litigation. Equally important and interesting, cancer was the disease within which the context of this discussion impressively took place.

Continued Shaping of the Regulatory Process for Consent

Beginning in the 1960's, several events occurred which significantly changed the practice and process of informed consent in therapeutic research. One of the most important events, and clearly of greatest significance with regard to cancer and other related therapeutic research, was the publication of Henry Beecher's paper in the New England Journal of Medicine in 1966.[37] Beecher, a clinical investigator and anesthesiologist at Harvard, assembled 22 recent research reports which he pulled from the peer reviewed medical literature that contained, in his view, clear violations of both patients' human rights and the recognized ethical principles of informed consent. Of note, several of the research reports which he described were specifically related to cancer clinical research. One such case was a published report regarding a young woman with metastatic melanoma. In this research study, the investigators described excising one of the melanoma lesions from the patient and transplanting it onto the patient's mother. Subsequently, serum was withdrawn from the mother and given to the patient in hopes of producing an immune mediated tumor response. The patient went on to die relatively quickly of widespread metastatic disease. Even more horrific, the mother subsequently died of metastatic melanoma approximately one year later. Another of Beecher's examples, although described without identifiers, clearly included the much publicized case of the Jewish Chronic Disease Hospital.[14] Researchers in this study, in an attempt to gain information relevant to organ transplantation, injected malignant cells from cancer patients into elderly and debilitated noncancer patients at the hospital. Again, both of these cancer clinical research reports were published in the peer-reviewed medical literature.

As a result of Beecher's cancer research examples, and the other reports described, subsequent public and medical community outcry led to regulations in the late 1960's and early 1970's which resulted in greatly increased scrutiny of Government-sponsored clinical research.[3,14,38] Clinical researchers themselves undoubtedly became more sensitive to the issues regarding the use of patients, including those with cancer and others, as research subjects. Other events, including the disclosure to the public regarding the United States Public Health Service Syphilis Studies (also known as the Tuskegee Syphilis Study)[1,3,39] as well as the Thalidomide experience and subsequent passage of the 1962 amendments to the Food, Drug, and Cosmetic Act,[40] also had great impact on the regulatory requirements for informed consent in clinical research. All of these events eventually led to the creation of the National Commission for the protection of human subjects in biomedical and behavioral research. The resulting recommendations of the National Commission led to the now required and pervasive practice of formalized institutional review of clinical research protocols and the use of the consent process as a means of protection of research subjects from potential harm.[4]

A SPECIAL CONSIDERATION IN INFORMED CONSENT: THE DILEMMA OF PHASE I TRIALS

Overall, the single largest group of consent forms reviewed by many IRB's, i.e., those used to convey information to potentially vulnerable patients making decisions about whether to become the subjects of research in clinical trials, are those employed in the cancer setting.[22] As well, and perhaps as a result, a significant proportion of the empiric research conducted examining the informed consent process has been in this setting.[23,24,25] Thus, it is in this setting where a great deal can be learned with regard to the current practice of informed consent in all therapeutic clinical trials, even those outside the context of cancer research.

Although difficult problems exist with regard to the informed consent process for all phases of clinical research, from an ethical perspective these difficulties are probably intensified in the earliest stages of the clinical trial spectrum. More specifically, it is within phase I cancer trials that many ethical dilemmas remain unresolved and where the general concerns about informed consent in therapeutic clinical trials become especially troubling and challenging.[4,23,41,42] Several of these dilemmas have arisen as a result of uncertainty regarding what the actual structure and outcome of the informed consent process should be for patients considering participation in these trials. Phase I trials typically involve patients with advanced (eventually life ending) disease in a research endeavor where the chance of meaningful objective therapeutic benefit has traditionally been described as being quite low. As a result of the dose escalation methods in these trials, a very specific dilemma is the relative ratio of toxicity and benefit for patients who participate.

Currently accepted phase I trial policy suggests that the goals of such research are to determine the toxicities and maximum-tolerated dose (MTD) of an investigational drug or drugs.[43,44] The toxic effects of a drug must be studied to determine if they are predictable, tolerable, and/or reversible. Based on dose-response information, it is believed that the greatest chance for tumor response occurs at the highest achievable dose. Phase I trials in oncology have traditionally involved a process of administering an investigational drug at very low-dose levels to initial cohorts of patients with refractory malignancies. Subsequently, through a process of dose escalation, with or without pharmacokinetic guidance,[45,46] later cohorts of patients are given higher doses of drug to eventually reach toxic levels, at which there is the greatest chance for therapeutic benefit. The standard process of dose escalation occurs through a conservative stepwise design that typically enrolls three initial patients. Thereafter, based on the amount of toxicity that may or may not develop, either the dose is escalated or additional patients are added to the cohort. It thus becomes necessary to give enough of any drug until the MTD is reached before being able to conclude that a drug has been adequately tested.

Overall, the chance of tumor response in phase I trials is low. In the four most comprehensive reviews, response rates of only 4% to 6% have been found.[47,48,49,50] Slightly more than half of these responses have occurred at 80% to 120% of the subsequently recommended dose for phase II trials, i.e., at or near the MTD. Thus, while some responses may occur in the larger population of cohorts treated at less toxic doses, the rates of response are higher as the MTD is approached. It is also important to note, and perhaps contrary to what many might believe, that the chance of fatal toxicity is low at approximately 0.5%.[48]

Further complicating this process is the need to adequately inform advanced cancer patients about these particular issues and then allow them to willingly and freely consent to participate in such studies. The complexities of the consent process for advanced cancer patients in phase I trials relate both to what degree such patients should be viewed as vulnerable, and to what extent a participating physician's own expectations and interests play a role in guiding patients to decide to participate. This unique form of therapeutic clinical research creates an intense environment of medical decision-making where, arguably, many patients may not benefit from the traditional informed consent process.

If patients were to participate in phase I trials solely for altruistic reasons, i.e., to help forward cancer research and potentially help future cancer patients, phase I trials would probably carry less ethical conflict. As well, this might imply that the traditional informed consent process might more readily achieve the desired ideal outcome of understanding of all elements of consent, including an understanding of the nature of phase I research and the alternatives to trial participation, as these less vulnerable patients would not necessarily be seeking benefit for themselves. However, the objective information available regarding the informed consent process for patients participating as research subjects in phase I trials tells us that altruism is not the primary motivating factor for patients participating in such clinical research. The available data also inform us that the current methods used to conduct the informed consent process within phase I trials may be inadequate.

Empiric Research on the Phase I Consent Process

In the first such study, Rodenhuis evaluated the quality of informed consent among patients with advanced cancer who were offered participation in a phase I trial.[51] In this study, the informed consent process consisted of three separate conversations taking place between patient, family and investigators (including both physicians and nurses). Following the three consent sessions, patients were surveyed regarding their attitude and motivations for participation. The majority of patients who gave their consent were motivated by hope for improvement of their condition, pressure exerted by relatives and friends, or simply because they felt they had "no choice". Some patients did mention the desire to contribute to the progress of medicine. The investigators conclude that encouragement by relatives or friends appears to be a powerful force in motivating patients to participate in phase I trials. In a similar but much smaller series of European advanced cancer patients, Willem and Sessa found corroborating results with regard to patient motivations for participation in phase I trials.[52]

Investigators at the University of Chicago conducted an in-depth survey study of twenty-seven cancer patients who had given informed consent to participate in phase I trials at their institution.[53] Concurrently, the oncologist identified by the surveyed patients as responsible for their care and consent were surveyed as well. Eighty five percent of patients decided to participate in a phase I trial for reasons of possible therapeutic benefit, 11% because of the advice or trust of physicians, and 4% because of family pressure. Ninety three percent said they understood all (33%) or most (60%) of the information provided to them about the trial in which they had decided to participate. Only 33% were able to state the purpose of the trial in which they were participating, with patients able to state the purpose of phase I trials as dose escalation or dose finding studies being more educated (p=0.01). Surveyed oncologists had wide ranging beliefs regarding expectations of possible benefits and toxicities for their patients participating in a phase I trial. The authors conclude that patients who participate in phase I trials are almost exclusively motivated by the hope of therapeutic benefit. Altruistic feelings, while perhaps present, appear to have a very limited role in motivating patients to participate in these trials. As well, cancer patients who participate in phase I trials appear to have an adequate self-perceived knowledge of the risks of investigational agents. However, much less than half the patients studied appeared to have an adequate understanding of the purpose of phase I trials as dose escalation or dose determination studies. Subsequent studies conducted by these investigators in a much larger series of subjects have found similar findings. In fact, in a larger series of subjects, quantifiable survey data show that patients may even be less aware of the research purposes of phase I trials, and are unable to recall alternatives to clinical trial participation, including palliative care or other non-experimental therapies.[54,55]

Tomamichel and colleagues conducted an analysis of the communication process involved in informed consent for cancer patients agreeing to participate in phase I trials.[56] The researchers performed a quantitative examination of information exchange by applying a communication model to taped conversations between cancer patients and physicians who were discussing whether to participate in a phase I trial. Three consecutive conversations in which the investigator responsible for phase I studies, the research nurse and the patient's relatives and friends participated were recorded. The authors concluded that the informed consent procedure was satisfactory from a quantitative point of view. Interestingly, they found that the most important items of information were acceptably communicated to patients. However, they also stated that greater attention should be paid to the indirect messages and implied criticism of patients to improve their participation in decision making. They also conclude that physicians should become more skillful in providing adequate information and to improve their methods of communication.

Yoder and colleagues conducted a prospective study involving entry and exit interviews of 37 advanced cancer patients participating in phase I trials.[57] Patients were interviewed at the time of making a decision to enter a phase I trial, and then subsequently when they came off the trial. They specifically sought to examine patients expectations in addition to their overall experiences from participation in a phase I trial. They found that patients expected slightly increased support from family members and received more support than expected. Perhaps not surprisingly, patients' expectations for tumor response and increased communication with their physician were not met. Their expectations were also not met with regard to improvement of symptoms such as fatigue, nausea, and vomiting and weight loss. They noted that one strong theme that emerged from the data was hope and optimism. They conclude that an issue that needs further exploration is the extent to which patients accurately understand information in the consent form and in the process itself. Findings also supported the importance of communication between the patient and family and all members of the health care team, and stress the importance of oncology nurses who may be able to mediate the flow of information between physicians and patients.

Japanese investigators conducted a similar study attempting to characterize the motivation, comprehension and expectations of patients who had given informed consent to participate in phase I trials at the National Cancer Center in Japan.[58] Prior to receiving any investigational agents, 33 subjects were given a multiple choice questionnaire, and 32 of the subjects completed the survey. Quite interestingly, 63% of subjects stated they did not expect any benefit from participation in the study but wished to participate any way. Only 19% of subjects were found to be motivated (in closed-ended questioning) to participate in phase I trials by the possibility of therapeutic benefit. Nine percent stated they were participating because it seemed a better choice than no treatment, and 6% mentioned altruistic reasons for participation. With closed ended questioning, most patients appeared to comprehend the major features of a phase I trial, namely its investigational nature, the unknown effects of the agent investigated, and the unclear benefit to themselves. As well, nearly 60% of the patients anticipated they might suffer severe or life threatening side effects from participation. As many as 43% of subjects were able to accurately indicate (again, in closed ended questioning) the research purpose of a phase I trial as a dose determination study. When questioned regarding their expectations, despite their responses with regard to motivations to participate in phase I trials, more than half the subjects indicated that there might be personal benefit to themselves. Overall, 42% agreed that there was no better choice than the phase I trial. Slightly more than 1/3 of the subjects (35%) believed that it was possible that their cancer could be cured. As well, 12 subjects fully expected to be cured as a result of participation in a phase I trial. The investigators found that older adults had slightly higher expectations of cure from participation in the phase I trial (although this did not reach statistical significance).

One disturbing finding from these studies is the potential discrepancy between what patients think they understand and what they may actually understand. For example, the University of Chicago study found that 90% of patients stated they understood all or most of the information provided to them about the phase I trial in which they had agreed to participate.[53] However, only approximately one-third of the patients could state the purpose of a phase I trial, and an even smaller proportion of patients could state the research purpose of phase I trials in a much larger study.[55] This discrepancy likely results from several factors, including inadequate informed consent. It may also lie in the methodologic difficulties of determining what a patient actually understands in relation to the information they have been given.

The results from these empiric studies strongly support the argument that the current process of obtaining informed consent for phase I trials may be inadequate to appropriately insure that advanced cancer patients understand both the nature of the research in which they are participating, and the alternatives to trial participation. In addition, despite recognizing the existence of their potential vulnerability, we do not know how that vulnerability effects an advanced cancer patient's ability to give what is otherwise perceived to be adequate informed consent. Further research will be required to better understand and delineate these issues and their importance on the informed consent process in this difficult and highly charged setting.

As well, innovative methodologies for both informed consent and phase I research should also be explored in order to improve the process from both a methodologic and ethical perspective. One example of this innovation includes dynamic consent forms that change and are modified as a trial progresses and new information is learned, an approach called 'cohort-specific informed consent'.[59] Another intriguing example would be to involve patients directly in discussions and decisions about dose escalation, i.e., allowing patients greater freedom than currently exists to choose their own dose.[60] Though this would raise some new dilemmas, this process might ensure that truly informed patients better understand the process of phase I trial methods and, in turn, this might permit patients to autonomously make their own decisions regarding their willingness to assume certain risks. Such research would undoubtedly benefit our knowledge of the informed consent process toward all phases of cancer research, and even toward other clinical research outside the cancer setting where potential therapeutic benefits may be similarly small or unlikely.

CONCLUSION

A strong commitment to the informed consent process remains an undeniable ethical obligation for investigators and others participating in clinical research, whether for cancer or other diseases. The impact of the cancer clinical research process itself on the shaping of current attitudes and practices regarding the informed consent process is significant. As well, current methodologies used in the early cancer clinical trial process, i.e., phase I trials, present important and challenging dilemmas which must be addressed, and from which much can be learned. Continued research on the informed consent process in phase I cancer trials has the potential to examine the very ethical boundaries of clinical research and to objectively illuminate what have often become speculative aspects of the doctor-patient communication process in this setting.

Supported in part by Grants from the American Cancer Society (PRTA-24) and a Career Development Award from the American Society of Clinical Oncology.

REFERENCES

1. Faden RR, Beauchamp TL, King NMP. *A history and theory of informed consent.* Oxford University Press; New York, 1986.

2. Applebaum PS, Lindz CN, Meisel A. *Informed consent: legal theory and clinical practice.* Oxford University Press; New York, 1987.

3. Levine RJ. *Ethics and regulation of clinical research.* 2nd Edition. Vurland and Schwarzenburg; Baltimore, 1986.

4. National Commission for the Protection of Human Subjects of Biomedical and Behavioral Research. Belmont Report; ethical principles and guidelines for the protection of human subjects of research. Publication number (05) 78-0012. USGPO, Washington, DC, 1978.

5. Freedman B, Fuks A, Weijer C. Demarcating Research in Treatment: a systematic approach for the analysis of the ethics of clinical research. Clin Res 40:655-660, 1992.

6. Bok S. Shading the truth in informed consent for clinical research. J Kennedy Inst Ethics 1995; 5:1-17.

7. Pelligrino ED. Beneficence, scientific autonomy, and self-interest: Ethical dilemmas in clinical research. Camb Q Health Ethics 1992; 1:361-369.

8. Jonsen AR, Siegler M, Winslade WJ. *Clinical ethics.* 3rd edition, p146-149. McGraw-Hill; New York, 1992.

9. Schaffner KF. Ethical problems in clinical trials. J Med Philos 1986; 11:297-315.

10. Markman M. The objective clinical scientist versus the advocate: A complex ethical and political dilemma facing cancer investigators and the public. Cancer Invest 1995; 13:324-326.

11. Elks ML. Conflict of interest and the physician-researcher. J Lab Clin Med 1995; 126:19-23.

12. Hammerschmidt DE. When commitments and interests conflict. J Lab Clin Med 1995; 126:5-6.

13. Levine RJ. Clinical trials and physicians as double agents. Yale J Biol Med 1992; 65:65-74.

14. Katz J. Experimentation with human beings. Russell Sage Foundation. New York, 1972.

15. Annas GJ: The changing landscape of human experimentation: Nuremberg, Helsinki, and beyond. J Law-Med 1992; 2:119-140.

16. The President's Commission for the Study of Ethical Problems in Medicine and Biomedical and Behavioral Research: Implementing human research regulations: The adequacy and uniformity of federal rules and their implementation. USGPO, publication number 040-000-00471-8, Washington, DC, 1983.

17. Epstein LC, Lasagna L. Obtaining informed consent, form or substance. Arch Intern Med 1969; 123:682-688.

18. Gray BH, Cooke RA, Tannebaum AS. Research involving human subjects. The performance of institutional review boards is assessed in this empirical study. Science 1978; 201:1094-1101.

19. Hammerschmidt DE, Keanse MA. Institutional review board review lacks impact on the readability of consent forms for research. Am J Med Sci 1992; 304:341-351.

20. Edgar H, Rothman DJ. The institutional review board and beyond: future challenges to the ethics of human experimentation. J Milb Q 1995; 73:489-506.

21. Redshaw ME, Harris A, Baum JD. Research ethics committee audit: differences between committees. J Med Ethics 1996; 22:78-82.

22. Goldman J, Katz MD. Inconsistency and institutional review boards. JAMA 1982; 248:197-202.

23. Daugherty CK, Ratain MJ, Siegler M. Ethical issues in the clinical research of cancer, in Cancer: Principles and Practice of Oncology. Devita VT Hellman S, Rosenberg SA (eds). J.P. Lippincott, Philadelphia PA. 5th ed., 1997; pp 534-542.

24. Kent G. Shared understandings for informed consent: the relevance of psychological research on the provision of information. Soc Sci Med 1996; 43:1517-1524.

25. Verheggen FWSM, van Wijmen FCB. Informed consent in clinical trials. Health Policy 1996; 36:131-153.

26. Katz J. *Human Experimentation and Human Rights.* St. Louis Univ Law Jour 1993; 38:7-54

27. Engelhardt HT. *The Foundations of Bioethics.* 2nd edition; pp 330-335. Oxford University Press, New York, 1996.

28. Jonas H. Philosophical reflections on experimenting with human subjects. In Paul A. Freund, ed., *Experimentation with Human Subjects.* George Brazilier; New York, 1969.

29. The final report of the president's advisory committee. *The Human Radiation Experiments.* Oxford University Press; New York, 1996 (ACHRE).

30. Lederer SE. *Subjected to Science: Human Experimentation in America Before the Second World War.* Johns Hopkins University Press; Baltimore, 1995.

31. Howard-Jones N. Human Experimentation in Historical and Ethical Perspectives. Soc Sci Med 1982; 16:1429-1448.

32. Salgo V. Leland Stanford Jr., the University Board of Trustees, 317 P. 2nd 170, 1957.

33. Katz J. *The Silent World of Doctor and Patient.* The Free Press; New York, 1984.

34. Obituary: PG Gebhard, 69, developer of the term "informed consent". New York Times, August 26, 1997.

35. ACHRE, p. 46-53

36. ACHRE, p. 53-67.

37. Beecher HK: Ethics in clinical research. N Engl J Med 1966; 274:1354-1360.

38. Rothman DJ: Ethics and human experimentation: Henry Beecher revisited. N Engl J Med 1987; 317:1195-1199.

39. Jones JH. *Bad Blood.* 2nd edition. Free press; New York, 1993.

40. ACHRE, p. 98-99.

41. Ratain MJ, Mick R, Schilsky R, Siegler M: Statistical and ethical issues in the design and conduct of phase I and II clinical trials of new anticancer agents. J Natl Cancer Inst 1993; 85:1637-1643.

42. Vanderpool HY. *The Ethics of Research Involving Human Subject: Facing the 21st Century.* p 306: University Publishing Group, Frederick, Maryland, 1996.

43. Simon RM: Clinical Trials in Cancer in Devita VT, Hellman S, Rosenberg SA (eds): *Principles and Practice of Oncology* (ed 5). Philadelphia, PA, Lippincott, pp 513-528, 1997.

44. Gordon NH, Williams JKV: Using toxicity grades and analysis of cancer phase I clinical trials. Stat Med 1992; 11:2063-2075.

45. Collins JM, Greishaber CK, Chabner BA: Pharmacologically guided phase I clinical trials based upon preclinical drug development. J Natl Cancer Inst 1990; 82:1321-1326.

46. Graham MA, Workman P: The impact of pharmacokinetically guided dose escalation strategies in phase I clinical trials: Critical evaluation and recommendations for future studies. Ann Oncol 1992; 3:339-347.

47. Von Hoff DD, Turner J: Response rates, duration of response, and dose response effect in phase I studies in antineoplastics. Invest New Drugs 1991; 9:115-122.

48. Decoster G, Stein G, Holdener EE: Responses and toxic deaths in phase I clinical trials. Ann Oncol 1990; 2:175-781.

49. Estey E, Hoth D, Wittes R, et al: Therapeutic responses in phase I trials of antineoplastic agents. Cancer Treat Rep 1986; 70:1105-1115.

50. Smith TL, Lee JJ, Kantarjian HM, et al: Design and results of phase I cancer clinical trials: 3 year experience at MD Anderson Cancer Center. J Clin Oncol 1996; 14:287-295.

51. Rodenhuis S, van-den Heuvel WJ, Annyas AA, Koops HS, Sleijfer DT, Mulder NH: Patient motivation and informed consent in a phase I study of an anticancer agent. Eur J Cancer Clin Oncol 1984; 20:457-62.

52. Willem Y, Sessa C: Informing patients about phase I trials-How should it be done? Aeta Oncol 1989; 28:106-107.

53. Daugherty CK, Ratain MJ, Grochowski E, Stocking C, Kodish E, Mick R, Siegler M: Perceptions of cancer patients and their physicians involved in phase I trials. J Clin Oncol 1995; 13:1062-1072.

54. Daugherty CK, Lyman K, Mick R, Siegler M, Ratain MJ: Differences in perceptions of goals, expectations, and level of informed consent in phase I clinical trials. Proc Amer Soc Clin Oncol 1996; 15:A352.

55. Daugherty CK, Kialbasa TA, Siegler M, Ratain MJ: Informed consent in clinical research: a study of cancer patient understanding of consent forms and alternatives of care in phase I clinical trials. Proc Amer Soc Clin Oncol 1997; 16:A188.

56. Tomamichiel M, Sessa C, Herzig S, de-Jong J, Pagani O, Willems Y, Cavalli F: Informed consent for phase I studies: Evaluation of quantity and quality of information provided to patients. Ann Oncol 1995; 6:321-323.

57. Yoder LH, O'Rourke TJ, Ethyre A, Spears DT: Expectations and experiences of patients with cancer participating in phase I clinical trials. Oncol Nurs Forum 1997; 24:891-896.

58. Itoh K, Sasaki Y, Fuji H, Ohtsu T, Wakita H, Igarashi T, Abe K: Patients in phase I trials of anti-cancer agents in Japan: Motivation, comprehension and expectations. Br J Cancer 1997; 76:107-113.

59. Freedman B: Cohort-specific consent: An honest approach to phase I cancer studies. IRB Rev Human Subjects Res 1990; 12:5-7.

60. Daugherty CK, Ratain MJ, Minami H, Banik DM, Vogelzang NJ, Stadler NJ, Siegler M: Study of cohort-specific consent and patient control in phase I cancer trials. J Clin Oncol 1998; 16:2305-2312.

8 THE ETHICAL LESSONS OF MANAGED CARE APPLIED TO CLINICAL TRIALS

Samuel Hellman, M.D.

INTRODUCTION

With increasing experience there have developed growing concerns with the ethical consequences of managed care. Some of these concerns are with the notion of rationing limited resources while others are with assuring timely appropriate care under the direction of a doctor of the patient's choosing. The resulting public and professional discussions have illuminated and emphasized the importance of patient rights and of the nature of the relationship between the patient and the health care provider. In this essay I shall try to extract the underlying ethical issues inherent in these concerns. I shall then apply them to another ethically troubling medical technique; the randomized clinical trial. I do this because while the concerns are similar, physician and public response is quite different; medical practitioners and the public are wary of managed care while physicians appear to embrace and the public accepts the use of randomized trials in the context of patient care.

MANAGED CARE

An apocryphal print shop is reported to have a sign next to the order counter offering:

Quality, Cost, Speed

Choose Only Two!!

This sign makes apparent the tension associated with trying to achieve high quality at low cost and at maximum speed. Today, there is a similar tense triad in medical care as we attempt to achieve superior, economical medical care that is equitably distributed. The Clinton administration proposal "The President's Health Security Plan" emphasized equity and cost control but many people worried about the maintenance of high quality. That plan has not come to fruition; rather, we have seen an explosion in private managed care. As such it is responsive to the marketplace with cost control being the main objective. It has been suggested that rather than managed care this is managed cost.

Managed care produces a second uncomfortable triad as well; a *manage a trois* of patient, doctor, and managed care organization quite different than the traditional bilateral doctor-patient relationship. The conflicts associated with both triads - quality, cost and equity; doctor, patient and managed care organization - are the root of public and professional concern. Many individual physicians as well as professional medical groups have registered concern as to how the doctor-patient relationship is affected by managed care. While we must attend to the difficulties of controlling cost, maintaining quality and fairly distributing health care, we must also be wary of the effect of interposing the managed care organization into the relationship between patient and doctor. In this new way to practice medicine, often the responsibility for husbanding limited resources resides in the treating physician thereby introducing an additional responsibility for the doctor. This - as well as requiring prior approval for referral and treatment - has resulted in changing the nature of the medical encounter.

While there is a growing acceptance of the need to control the rate of rise of medical expenditures there does not appear to be consensus on how this is to be accomplished. Agreement in general terms dissolves when it is applied to individual patient care. The public is also uneasy with explicitly recognizing medical rationing. Most disconcerting for both doctors and patients is the notion that the physician should be the rationing agent.[1] Physicians will be needed as expert consultants but the decisions regarding the relative value of high-cost low yield diagnostic procedures, investments in expensive procedures for the elderly, palliative care and many other issues require community more than medical judgment. It is only such communally determined principles delineating the rights and responsibilities of individuals that can ensure that difficult rationing decisions are consonant with societal values.

Managed care appears to some as more likely than fee-for-service medicine, with a cost-based reimbursement system, to control costs and to limit over-utilization and overcharging. In the past because the practice of medicine was relatively unconstrained by cost considerations, therapeutic efficacy – the capacity to produce a desired effect – was valued regardless of expense. In contrast, the competition between various care providers emphasizes efficiency – efficacy as a function of cost – rather than efficacy alone. While this may result in limiting medical utilization, it raises concerns as to the choices, extent, and most importantly, the relevant criteria used to determine the efficient use of resources. Society must provide guidelines that balance efficacy and efficiency to achieve satisfactory quality, quantity and distribution of health care. The physician in dealing with an individual patient must then provide a program that maximizes that individual patient's benefits within these socially defined limits. Inherent in most of the public concerns with managed care is the choice of a personal physician. This is because of both perceived medical expertise and the loyal patient advocacy expected of the physician. Preserving the valuable doctor-patient relationship requires separating the primary responsibility of the individual physician to the patient being cared for from the responsibility for controlling health care costs. Bedside rationing is bad for the doctor, the patient, and the community.

Personal Care

The physician in the doctor-patient relationship is expected to provide personal care requiring that patient is seen as an individual rather than as a member of a group of patients with similar characteristics. It is expected that the care is fashioned to meet the individual determinants of that patient's illness, other medical conditions, attitudes, beliefs and preferences.[1] If, in the managed care organization, the physician is also asked to husband the group's resources. either by limiting the pool of funds available for the care of a panel of patients or by compensating the physician according to the extent of resource utilization, then the physician can no longer be concerned only with maximizing that patient's benefits. Furthermore, even treatment guidelines for groups of patients with similar traits currently being promulgated as a method to ensure good care may discourage personal care tailored to the individual. Justice Charles Fried, then of the Harvard Law School and now of the Massachusetts Supreme Judicial Court, worried more than 20 years ago that the personal care inherent in the doctor-patient relationship would be replaced by "the physician as agent of an efficient health care delivery system."[2] That concern seems even more pressing today.

Not only does the physician act as double agent[3] when responsible for serving both the patient's best interests and parsimony, he or she is also, in part, a secret agent. The doctor's duty to the managed care organization to constrain cost is usually unknown by if not hidden from the patient. There are 'gag' rules in some plans that specifically prohibit the physician from revealing the general financial arrangements, all the treatment options, and the particular pecuniary implications associated with treatment decisions. There have always been some societal restrictions limiting the physician from being completely the patient's agent even in the traditional relationship. Examples of this are the required reporting of certain diseases or wounds caused in a suspicious fashion. These exceptions are limited, explicit and open, providing boundaries within which the physician is expected to serve only the patient's best interests.

It does not appear that informed consent is given by the patient to any modification of physician loyalty in the managed care doctor-patient relationship. Even if the patient accedes to a modified doctor-patient relationship in managed care, the physician should have great difficulty in participating in a situation that requires such divided loyalties. This conflict is the basis of much of physician concern with practicing in many managed care settings. The basis of medicine as a profession requires that the physician's efforts are devoted to serve the patient's best interests. This is not to suggest that in fee-for-service medicine physician behavior is not potentially affected by financial considerations. In the past both patients and doctors understood that the more physicians did the more they were rewarded. The patient expected and professional code required that the doctor ignore these pecuniary considerations and act only in the patient's best interest. In contrast, having physicians responsible for the financial success of the managed care organization in the context of individual patient care results in a new trilateral arrangement which prevents the assurance of the undivided loyalty of the doctor to the individual patient. The President in his 1998 State Of The Union Address recognized the potential endangerment of patient rights in health care. Because of concern that they may be modified by managed care he promulgated that legislation be enacted to assure the rights that all therapeutic options are presented and that patients may choose a personal physician.

We can conclude from this discussion that there is a right to some level of health care although the extent of the services provided is undefined. Rationing is necessary but is better placed with the community rather than as a part of the doctor-patient relationship. Pertinent to the further discussion is identifying the individual's rights in health care. These rights include:

1) Personal care, a care plan reflecting that patient as an individual.
2) Loyalty, the physician - bound by the precepts of the profession- should serve the patient's interests before any other.
3) Informed consent, while there may be differences in the level of detail provided, the patient must be sufficiently informed to make an autonomous decision.
4) Honesty the physician must reveal all treatment alternatives and indicate potential conflicts of interest.

Loyalty to the patient, fidelity to professional obligations and honesty, all of which must be based on the fundamental obligation of beneficence are the expected principles of the doctor-patient relationship to be applied to a personal plan of care.

RANDOMIZED CLINICAL TRIALS

Let us now consider the application of these concepts to the randomized clinical trial. As is often done in medicine let's begin with an actual case, one which was presented to me in an Ethics Rounds, in order to explore how these principles apply to this practice of clinical investigation.[4]

Case Presentation

A 29 year old women discovered a mass in her left breast. A mammogram was unremarkable but biopsy revealed a 1.5 cm cancer and removal of the axillary lymph nodes revealed that two of thirteen lymph nodes were involved with tumor.

The physician spent ninety minutes with the patient and her husband explaining the nature of her breast cancer. He indicated that the real question for her was not whether she should receive chemotherapy but rather what type should be administered. He reviewed the standard therapy but suggested that, despite the small size of the lesion, there were some adverse factors in her particular case. He stated that given her disease and her age many oncologists would urge more aggressive treatment than standard chemotherapy. If she were to consider such aggressive treatment he stated that there was a protocol for such treatment. He explained the rationale for more intensive therapy, but that at this point there was no proof that this intensive treatment was more effective. The patient and her husband wanted to consider the more aggressive chemotherapy but also to discuss fertility issues. After ninety minutes of discussion of both the effects of the drugs on fertility as well as the differences between the conventional and aggressive treatment the patient and her husband left to consider the options. A few days later the nurse practitioner called the patient to ask whether there were any questions about the protocol. The patient seemed quite confused asking if the nurse practitioner was referring to some kind of "experimental treatments." The nurse practitioner tried to explained the rationale for conducting a clinical trial. The patient seemed shocked by the idea of considering an experimental treatment.

That evening the patient's husband called quite upset to say that neither he nor the patient had realized that the more aggressive chemotherapy was a part of a randomized trial until told by the nurse practitioner. The physician apologized for not making it clear and explained again the trial and the randomization. The husband said that the patient would not be randomized but wanted to receive the aggressive treatment. The physician indicated that he could not give her that aggressive chemotherapy 'off protocol'. The patient's husband insisted that if more intensive therapy was best that is what he wanted his wife to have. The physician explained that oncologists had reason think that the new treatment might be better but they had no scientific proof and that the trial was an attempt to get that proof. Without the proof the physician claimed that he could not give them chemotherapy 'off protocol'. The husband insisted that from the extensive discussions both he and his wife determined that the physician favored this treatment. There then ensued a discussion of the rationale for randomized trials and the difference between suspecting that something is better and proving it. After this, the husband reemphasized that his wife would not participate in a randomized trial but wanted the most intensive therapy.

Application of the Lessons of Managed Care

The previous discussions of managed care elucidated the principles of the doctor-patient relationship to be observed in any medical encounter. The patient should expect from the physician: personal care, honesty, fidelity and loyalty. Implicit in the current doctor patient relationship is also the recognition of the vulnerability of the patient and the physician's role to assure her interests are the basis for the management plan. Concern with the dual responsibility to the managed care organization and to the patient is mirrored in the relationship of the personal physician with scientific investigation. The patient expects an individually designed treatment program that requires her autonomous assent. How consistent is the case presented with these principles?

While the physician spent a great deal of time with the patient and her husband and he recognized the young age and poor prognostic markers, it appears that personal care is compromised in that she is to be treated as a member of an experimental group rather than have a treatment crafted to her individual circumstances. Randomization does not assure that she will get the aggressive treatment and, while acceptable medical practice permits, the physician refuses to treat the patient 'off protocol' thereby questioning his loyalty to the patient. This also suggests some element of coercion since participation in the trial is offered as the only way to get the more intensive therapy. The doctor has been honest but what about his fidelity to his obligations as a physician? The patient and her husband have deduced from the discussion that the doctor favors the aggressive treatment. Both fidelity to his professional responsibility and loyalty to the patient should require his offering treatment in the manner he believes most appropriate. It does not require formal scientific proof. While uncertain, he believes it is better and she and her husband desire it. He admits that while he favors aggressive treatment, the study is being done to determine whether this opinion can be substantiated. Of course even a positive result does not settle the issue with certainty, rather it reduces the likelihood that any difference observed is due to chance.

The patient is in a dependent vulnerable position and the physician is expected to act as her agent providing the treatment that he favors and she desires.[5] Even if the aggressive treatment has not been proven to be superior, she has not come for proof, she came for his expert opinion. While not the subject of this discussion surely states of knowledge are not binary; knowing with certainty or complete ignorance. There are many intermediary positions and it is these that obtain in most medical decisions. All patients are different – requiring application of trial results and other knowledge to the specific patient. The physician has such an intermediate position and has indicated it to her, as he should. Now he should implement the personal care appropriate to this patient considering her unique medical circumstances as well as her preferences. Making knowing and ignorance the only alternatives allows the physician a way of avoiding individual patient responsibility. It may be considered analogous to a 'gag' rule since it limits patient information and options. Whether in clinical trials or managed care the patient expects the physician to act as her advocate. In trials and managed care, agreement with goals in general fails to reflect the difficulties in their implementation in individual patient care.

DIFFERING RESPONSES TO SIMILAR ISSUES

These infringements on the essentials of the doctor patient relationship in trials are viewed quite differently than those occurring in managed care; they are accepted in trials and rejected in managed care. This is the result of the attitudes of both the medical profession and the public. For the profession, managed care and cost control threaten to diminish the role and autonomy of the physician, while clinical trials increase the knowledge and status of the physician. Indeed the appellation physician-scientist confers this more exalted station. Fear of the return to anecdotal unscientific medicine is offered as sufficient justification for the use of randomized trials as if this is the only scientific method for acquiring knowledge and informed consent assures patient autonomy. For the patient, managed care means rationing, reduced trust in the doctor, and loss of autonomy. The inherent trust in the physician allows a positive attitude toward trials while the profession's concerns with managed care reinforce patient concerns. Participation in a trial may be troubling but it is balanced by the assurances of the doctor that participation in a trial will not compromise care. It is concern about these assurances that caused the patient presented to be unwilling to participate. Both managed care and randomized clinical trials balance patient rights with utilitarian concerns but these are believed to be primarily pecuniary in managed care while clinical trials increase knowledge. The difference in patient acceptance may depend on the values placed on these goals. It may also have to do with different levels of trust placed by the patient in the care provider in these different settings. Patients appear to trust doctors of their choosing while being suspicious of managed care organizations. But both managed care and clinical trials raise questions of: competing physician interests, secrecy, coercion, personal care, patient autonomy, and beneficence. From both of these troubling practices a principle that will serve us well is to separate the role of physician from that of providing societal, group or personal gain. Not only is bedside rationing a conflict of interest, so too is that of the personal physician as a trialist.

CONCLUSION

It may be argued that this discussion idealizes the physician and his or her relationship to the patient. While this may be the case, it is consistent with the current incarnations of the Hippocratic Oath, the World Medical Association's Declaration of Helsinki, and the criticisms of managed care. Perhaps underlying the ambivalence of the profession is its acceptance of dual responsibilities placed on the physician; that care of the individual patient must be considered in the context of the public good. Then we should be explicit enumerating and carefully describing the constraints and priorities guiding these different responsibilities if we are to avoid a 'slippery slope' problem. While I am convinced that the profession is best served by insulating the doctor when dealing with the individual patient from other responsibilities, if this is not to be the case it seems a poor idea to have dual goals without making them clear to the individual patient, the public, and the profession.

REFERENCES

1. Hellman S. The patient and the public good. Nature Medicine 1995; 1:400-402.

2. Fried C. Rights and health care - beyond equity and efficiency. N Eng J Med 1975;293:241-45.

3. Angell M. The doctor as a double agent. Kennedy Inst Ethics J 1993; 3:279-286.

4. Emanuel EJ, Patterson WB. Ethics of randomized clinical trials. Journal Clin Oncol 1998; 16:365-371.

5. Hellman S, Hellman D. Of mice but not men. Problems of the randomized clinical trial. N Engl J Med 199 1;324:1585-1589.

9 KIDS AND CANCER: ETHICAL ISSUES IN TREATING THE PEDIATRIC ONCOLOGY PATIENT

Sarah E. Friebert, M.D.
Eric D. Kodish, M.D.

CASE REPORT 1

SC was 14 years old when she was diagnosed with a Ewing's sarcoma of the left distal femur, metastatic to both lungs. She had been in her usual state of good health until three months prior to admission, when she developed intermittent leg pain near her knee. Initially the pain did not interrupt her normal activities, but over the ensuing two months, the pain worsened and began to awaken her at night. She also noticed the onset of pain on inspiration, without dyspnea or hemoptysis. SC denied any constitutional symptoms such as fever or weight loss. Two weeks prior to admission, an MRI demonstrated a left leg mass. Open biopsy confirmed Ewing's sarcoma, and a CT scan of the chest revealed multiple bilateral pulmonary lesions.

SC was the youngest of three children. She was born in Australia, and moved here with her family at seven years of age. Prior to her illness, SC was an excellent student who was well-liked and participated in many extracurricular activities.

Before SC was informed, her parents were told about the biopsy and CT scan results in a private setting. Both parents were devastated by the news and quickly agreed that SC should not be told. They demanded that the health care team refrain from disclosing the diagnosis to SC, suggesting instead that she be told she had an infection that had spread to her lungs. Despite numerous attempts over several days, the physicians and nurses caring for SC could not persuade her parents to permit SC to be informed of her diagnosis.

INTRODUCTION

The basic principles guiding the ethical practice of pediatrics are identical to those in adult medicine. These include the "big four": respect for persons, beneficence, nonmaleficence, and justice. In addition, proportionality, or an analysis of the benefits versus the burdens of a particular situation or treatment, becomes a key fifth element in clinical ethics. Sources of ethical guidance are also consistent across age; most practitioners rely on principles, casuistry (case-based ethical formulation), and a "care perspective," a concept that compels the provider to care for a patient as a unique individual with a view toward preserving existing relationships.[1]

Despite these similarities, however, pediatric ethics is necessarily a separate discipline. As the case above illustrates, not only are children different from adults in terms of age, but ethical practice is also different within the specialized world of pediatric oncology. Here, the challenges of dealing with serious or terminal illness in the context of a research-oriented tertiary care center create unique ethical issues worthy of closer investigation. This chapter will start by reviewing the need to consider pediatric ethical issues separately, the problem of competence in children, and general medical decision making in pediatrics. We will then examine pediatric oncology in detail, turning our attention to an in-depth look at information disclosure and at children as research subjects. Following this, we will discuss particular aspects of the field fraught with ethical dilemmas: withdrawal/withholding of treatment, DNR/CPR in children, physician-assisted suicide/euthanasia, terminal sedation, and end-of-life care for children, including palliative and hospice care. We hope to reveal the complexity of the ethical issues in pediatric oncology and to offer current thoughts on caring for seriously ill children.

What Makes Children Different

In several respects which are particularly relevant to clinical ethics, children are not simply small adults. First, the diseases which afflict children differ in number, type, and manifestations from those which befall adults. Second, children are in the throes of developing decision-making capacity throughout childhood. Three broad types of capacities are necessary for decision-making competence: understanding information and ability to communicate that understanding; reasoning and deliberation; and possession and application of a set of values or conception of the good.[2] Children may "have a right to be treated as developing persons, as persons with a developing capacity for rationality, autonomy, and participation in health-care decision making."[3] At any given age, however, they may possess none, some, or all of the capacities necessary to participate in their own health care depending upon their maturity level.

Third, children possess numerous physical and cognitive differences which make specific research with children absolutely imperative. Dramatic changes in overall body growth, proportion, composition, and physiology occur throughout childhood, alongside unique fears, anxieties and perceived bodily threat.[4] Together, these factors mandate separate research efforts on pediatric subjects.

Finally, the most compelling clinical difference between children and adults is the simple maxim, held by caregivers and families alike, that children are not supposed to develop cancer, become seriously ill, or die. Children represent the hope of the future and the promise of lives yet unlived. They are innocent beings who have done nothing to contribute to their own ill health. For these reasons, the diagnosis of cancer in a child magnifies all the attendant issues of cruelty, unfairness, and guilt that accompany the diagnosis of cancer in adults.[5]

What Makes Pediatric Ethics Different

The ethical practice of medicine involves a set of responsibilities which are the same for all physicians, namely providing maximum benefit while refraining from harm. The goals of medical intervention are also universal beyond specialty, and include restoration of health, relief of symptoms, restoration of impaired fuction, and saving and/or prolonging life.

Above and beyond these general principles, pediatrics entails a unique approach. Pediatric health care providers are entrusted with the care of vulnerable patients, whose development and future productivity have the potential to be significantly shaped through encounters with the medical profession. Additionally, children do not live in isolation, and caring for them requires interaction with the child's family and environment.[6] This point is particularly salient in the case of SC, whose interaction with her health care team was severely curtailed by her parents' request. Pediatricians must often be guided by surrogate decision making. Of necessity, these special responsibilities of pediatric providers demand separate consideration of ethical issues in treating pediatric patients, particularly those with life-threatening illnesses such as cancer.

MEDICAL DECISION MAKING FOR CHILDREN

The application of ethical principles to decision making for children in medical situations is often likened to that of incompetent adults. Here, medical decisions are made by surrogates who act through one of several mechanisms: legal/procedural means (i.e., using advance directives); subjective standards determined by previous competent declarations (i.e., substituted judgment); or objective standards of a reasonable person (the best interest standard). The framework for these decisions is justified by the principles of patient self-determination and well being.

Surrogate Decision Making

Standards

Historically, children have been declared legally and ethically incompetent to participate in decisions about their own health care.   Except for certain circumstances involving mature or emancipated minors (see below), decisions regarding health care for children under age eighteen are made by surrogate decision makers, usually parents. The standard for surrogates has generally been to rely more on best interest guidelines and to act toward promoting the well-being of the child instead of following legal/procedural or subjective standards. While a full discussion of competence is beyond the scope of this chapter, several contrasts between adult and pediatric decision making are worth reviewing.

Underlying Tenets of Competence

One approach holds that because children have never possessed competence, they are incapable of formulating advance directives on their own, nor have they developed sufficiently mature aims and values to limit the choices made by their surrogates.[7]   Logically, it follows from this line of reasoning that substituted judgment also cannot apply to decision making if competence was never achieved. This view places severe limitations on children's ability to participate in their own health care and will be explored in more detail later.

A second tenet upholding surrogate decision making involves protection of future autonomy.   This position holds that for children, fulfillment of self-determination lies in protection and promotion of the capacity to develop autonomy, rather than in making decisions for themselves or in having decisions made by others in accordance with their current aims and values. Third, children may not possess the necessary understanding of the impact of treatment alternatives on life. Fourth, the determination of "well-being" for children is quite different from that of adults. For children, well-being depends more on objective conditions necessary to foster future development and opportunities; for adults, the determination rests more on current individual preferences.   In other words, children may not possess sufficient forward-thinking ability to look out for their own best interests. Fifth, competence for children is a threshold concept: its possession must be proven to exist rather than be removed, as is the case for adults.   Sixth, determination of competence is different for children in that the process is parent- as well as patient-centered. In fact, an additional prong in the decision-making process is occasionally described, representing the parent interest in making decisions about a child's welfare.[8]

Some ethicists believe that standards of competence in children should be higher than in adults. A determination of competence should be based on the child's reasoning process, not just his/her ability to come to the "correct" decision. If the consequences of the child's decision involve adverse outcomes, it should be necessary to prove with great certainty that the child possesses a higher level of decision-making capacity.[9] As is true for adults, competence to accept treatment does not equal competence to refuse. At present, there exists no legal mechanism to rebut the presumption of incompetence in children.

In pediatrics, several situations exist in which lack of parental or surrogate consent would discourage treatment that is otherwise important to a child's well being (such as treatment for sexually transmitted diseases or substance abuse). For these cases, emancipated minor or mature minor statutes have been enacted in most states to allow children to bypass surrogate decision making. Such statutes make it difficult to defend any general declaration that all minors are incompetent in health-care decision making, since some minors are exempt through these rules.

Parental Authority

Traditionally, parents maintain surrogate medical decision-making authority for their minor, incompetent children. Parental authority derives from several schools of thought.[10] According to utilitarian theory, parents should maintain control over treatment choices because they must bear the consequences of decisions made for their children. While keeping the locus of control within the family, this approach has the potential to saddle parents with guilt should their decision not lead to a desired outcome. A rights-based approach holds that parents have the right to raise their children according to their own standards and values. This approach holds as long as parental values are not seen as harmful to the best interests of the child.

Under the zone of discretion idea, children are incapable of deciding for themselves, and parents will do the best job because they love their children and want what's best for them. However, parents possess no independent rights to decide or enforce their decisions if their decision is clearly outside a reasonable zone of discretion and is inconsistent with the best interests of their child. Lastly, the zone of privacy theory describes the family as a social institution whose job is to foster intimacy and provide privacy. Within this context, decisions concerning incompetent vulnerable members may be made for the good of the child or the good of the social construct (the family) without external review.

Perhaps the most compelling argument for parental authority, though, is the common observation that children usually prefer that parents decide. Such a child-centered view protects the integrity of the family unit by respecting the child's wishes at the same time that surrogate decision making is employed.

Special Features of Medical Decision Making for Children

Regardless of the theory employed to justify it, the ethical practice of surrogate decision making has the potential to be extremely complex. To begin with, the patient may be too young or immature to formulate preferences or make judgments about well-being at the outset of a treatment plan or alliance, but as maturity increases, the child's preferences and decisions may conflict with preexisting adult preferences. The nature of the relationship with the medical system must, therefore, be malleable and adaptable to change.

In addition, though parents clearly have extensive authority over the child/patient, this authority is not absolute and its legal boundaries remain ill-defined. The patient may have siblings for whose well-being the parents are equally responsible; potential conflict may arise when the needs of siblings interfere with or supercede those of the child in medical therapy. A further confounding factor is the difficulty of predicting adult values, preferences and quality of life from childhood.

Lastly, and perhaps most importantly, children represent the hope of the future. Medical care decisions and health policy have far-reaching impact in terms of number of life years and amount of productivity saved by curing children of cancer and other life-threatening illnesses. In actual practice, therefore, pediatric providers function as advocates and include children in health care decisions to the extent that they are able, rather than selecting an arbitrary competence threshold level or adhering strictly to a theory of surrogate decision making.[11]

THE CULTURE OF PEDIATRIC ONCOLOGY

Having begun our discussion by examining ethical principles as applied to pediatric practice in more general terms, we now turn our focus to the specialized milieu of pediatric oncology.

Multidisciplinary Approach

Unlike many medical specialties, pediatric oncology is practiced almost exclusively in tertiary care centers composed of highly-trained staff and well-equipped facilities to ensure the best care available for children with cancer and their families. In fact, research has repeatedly shown that pediatric cancer patients enjoy better outcomes when their care is coordinated through one of these comprehensive centers.[12] Hands-on care is provided by a multidisciplinary team approach: "Every parent, medical staff member and psychosocial professional involved in the care of the child should be responsible for cooperating in the child's best interest. Everyone must work together toward the common goal of curing the cancer and minimizing its medical and psychosocial side-effects."[13]

Because there are multiple professionals involved in each child's care, honesty and open communication are the cornerstones of success in this model. Since information does not consistently come from a single source, the potential for communication imbroglios to occur is high. The only remedy is to maximize the therapeutic relationship in all directions of the child-parent-doctor triangle, as depicted in Figure 1.

Figure 1: Patient/Parent/Medical Team Interaction in Pediatric Oncology

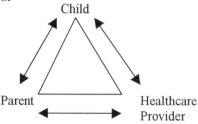

Reevaluating Competence

An essential component of a successful therapeutic relationship in pediatric oncology is the notion that the child must actively participate in his or her medical decision making in this model. Treatment of childhood cancer necessitates long and usually grueling treatment protocols involving great sacrifices of time, resources, energy, and normal daily activities (such as school). These treatment schemes are only successful to the extent that the child is an active, willing participant and that his or her decisions and feelings are respected to the largest degree possible. Respect for the child as an active participant stems from the general recognition that "involving patients, whether children or adults, in decisions about their treatment often promotes their well-being by increasing their level of compliance in cooperating with the caregiver, thereby enhancing the effectiveness of the treatment."[14]

In this context, the assessment of competence for the child with cancer becomes more multifactorial. Including the child in decisions about his or her treatment involves matching the capacity of the particular minor at a particular time under the particular conditions which exist with the demands of the particular task involved. This type of assessment obligates caregivers to be more invested and observant. Explanations of treatments must be offered in terms that families and patients can understand since more involved decision making is required. The treatment itself may have complex and similar but competing alternatives for any given condition; grasping these subtleties may require more understanding and reasoning than when one simpler, more standard, lower-risk and clearly beneficial treatment exists.[15] Thus, while straightforward surrogate decision making is unlikely to be beneficial for the pediatric oncology patient, the complexity of treatment necessitates increased involvement and ongoing assessment on the part of the caregiving team.

ETHICAL ISSUES IN PEDIATRIC CANCER CARE

The unique culture of pediatric oncology raises several areas of ethical concern worthy of more detailed analysis. These issues may be viewed on a chronologic continuum which begins with discussion of the initial diagnosis and treatment plan with the patient and family, extends to consideration of appropriate disclosure of information, involves potential enrollment in research initiatives, and concludes with issues surrounding end-of-life care. Children as research subjects opens the door for discussion of several key concepts, including informed consent and its terminology, assent of the child, ethical recruitment practices (particularly consent forms) and justifications, psychological factors affecting research participation, and ethical objections to children as research subjects. Each of these areas will be considered in more detail.

Initial Discussion with the Patient and Family

The importance of the initial discussion between the health care team and the patient and family cannot be overemphasized. Few single interactions in medicine have such power or potential for long-lasting effect. The diagnosis discussion establishes the degree of trust in and cooperation with the health care team, and sets the tone for most, if not all, future encounters with the family.

Delivery of bad news is a skill which is poorly taught in most formal health care curricula. In fact, some argue that the skills of a compassionate health care provider cannot be taught – they are either inherently possessed or sorely lacking. Nevertheless, various characteristics of the informer are identifiable and even quantifiable in their importance during the initial interaction with the family. These include: competence, self-confidence, warmth and genuine interest in the patient and family, ability to listen, patience with and acceptance of negative responses to information offered, tolerance of expression of emotion, sensitivity to feeling states, ability to be honest and direct, sound clinical judgment, and use of language understandable to parents and patients.[16]

In addition to skillful presentation of information, the health care team must give careful thought to the people who should attend the initial series of discussions. Children themselves should not be excluded from these encounters, unless they specify that they do not want to be included. Even very young children are capable of understanding what is happening to their bodies and what they will be asked to do during treatment, if the information is presented in a developmentally-appropriate fashion. Along with the affected child, every effort must be made to include those family members or support people most pertinent to the child's world. This may occasionally necessitate a delay in the discussion to allow support people to arrive, or result in adversarial parties being present together, as in divorced parents. Health care providers are obliged to remember that temporary inconvenience for them may result in a more informed and cohesive support network capable of providing qualtiy care for the child over the long haul.

Disclosure of Information

A key issue in the initial diagnosis talk is the degree of disclosure of information from the health care team. Pediatric oncology has shifted away from the paternalistic tendencies of past conversations of this sort, in which patients and families were not fully informed about the diagnosis, treatment plan, and prognosis. A number of early studies helped destroy the shield-and-protect paradigm which dominated early provider-patient interactions. As a typical example, Spinetta and Maloney demonstrated that children with leukemia as young as four years were well aware of their diagnoses and went so far as to try to protect their parents from harm or sadness by keeping silent about their knowledge.[17]

No published data has yet shown that honest disclosure of information is harmful to children. In fact, the opposite appears to be true: awareness of the full scope of the illness may actually produce less anxiety than receiving partial or no information.[18,19] Disclosure of pertinent information in an age- sensitive manner has actually been shown to prevent isolation, confusion, fear and stigmatization.[20] Most practitioners who are not honest with their pediatric patients have learned the hard way that children eventually discover the truth in most cases. When this happens, truthfulness is undermined and presents a substantial barrier to trust in the provider-patient relationship. Such arguments might be used to good effect in cases such as ours described at the beginning of this chapter.

There is a potential down-side to full disclosure of information in the pediatric oncology setting. It involves the fear that families will be overwhelmed by the amount of information presented at diagnosis and will be unable to process the information efficiently or completely. In other words, disclosure may paradoxically impair the exercise of autonomy by causing inability to prioritize. One response to this fear has been to provide titrated information -- that is, giving information in small bytes over an extended period of time, partitioned at the discretion of the health care provider. Ethically, this approach may be problematic because it relies on unjustified paternalism in the service of nonmaleficence. Such paternalism can be avoided by the astute clinician who uses good listening skills to allow the disclosure to be guided by signals from the patient and family.

Pediatric oncology providers must realize that the announcement of a potentially fatal disorder necessarily entails a grieving process for the loss of normality or the anticipated death of the child. Reaction by the family to this type of pronouncement predictably results in initial shock, followed by emotional disorganization and struggle to assimilate the information. Fortunately, the usual result is the development or uncovering of adequate coping mechanisms which allow children and families to continue to function. Provided frightening diagnostic information is offered by informers possessing the above-mentioned characteristics, families can be expected to adopt adquate coping styles relatively quickly. Oncology professionals may fear that such unadulterated disclosure may detract from the caregiver-parent/patient relationship, but research suggests this is not the case.[21]

Children as Research Subjects

Pediatric oncology is unique as a medical discipline in its heavy reliance on research protocols in the provision of patient care. In contrast to adult patients, most children in the United States who are diagnosed with cancer are treated at tertiary care centers on protocols designed by one of two major cooperative cancer groups, either the Pediatric Oncology Group (POG) or the Children's Cancer Group (CCG). While these protocols represent the standard of care, their use nonetheless constitutes research; participation must, therefore, be contingent upon informed consent.

The principles discussed below also apply to children with refractory or relapsed disease who are offered Phase I or Phase II clinical trial participation. An in-depth discussion of the ethics of Phase I and II trials will not be explored herein except to say that clinicians enrolling patients on these protocols need to strike a careful balance between the role of patient advocate and the role of researcher. Once again, open communication, along with an unbiased presentation of the available data, is the best defense against potential conflict.

The Doctrine of Informed Consent

Though a full discussion of informed consent is beyond the scope of this chapter, a basic discussion of its terminology and applicability to pediatrics is appropriate here. Briefly, the unacceptable paternalism which defined traditional medical practice earlier in this century led to the creation of the doctrine of informed consent to improve patient autonomy in medical decision making. Essential components of true informed consent are disclosure, understanding, voluntariness and competence. The ethical principle underlying the doctrine is respect for persons which is carried out through provision of information relevant to the exercise of decision-making rights.[22] For adults, benefit/burden assessment of a medical decision is determined by individual self-determination, not by society or public policy. The primary ethical underpinning is autonomy.

In contrast, informed consent in pediatric oncology actually amounts to "second-party consent."[23] Since children are deemed incompetent to make their own benefit/burden judgments, the ethical principles of nonmaleficence and beneficence take precedence over autonomy. The components of informed consent must also be analyzed carefully. Voluntariness, for instance, may be compromised in pediatric patients who tend to have an external locus of control and react strongly to authority figures, whether positively or negatively. Similarly, understanding and disclosure are heavily influenced by age-appropriate presentation of the pertinent information.[24] The bottom line again focuses on the necessites of participating in ongoing dialogue and of eliciting true understanding on the part of patients and families.

The Terminology of Informed Consent

Careful attention to language is paramount to obtaining true informed consent in both the practice and the research setting.

"Permission" specifically means what one person is capable of doing for another. On the other hand, "consent" entails what a person does autonomously. In pediatrics, consent actually amounts to authorization under the age of fourteen years, reflecting the assumption that parents are the most authentic spokespeople for their children. Generally speaking, children are capable of consent after age fourteen -- they have been shown to possess full decisional capacity and flexible thinking after attainment of Piaget's formal operations stage (at 11-13 years).[25,26] "Assent" refers to child agreement with the proposed treatment. Although not legally valid, assent respects children as persons with developing capacities for participation in health-care decision making. The term "coercion" describes an essentially paternalistic act of forcing participation in treatment or research; such an act may only be justifiable if the harm prevented by coercing participation is greater than the harm incurred by lack of participation. Such situations are extremely rare, and many ethicists argue that coercion is never justifiable in the research setting.

An earlier term, "proxy consent," describes the situation in which parents or guardians make all decisions in concert with health care providers. Largely due to the work of William Bartholome, this term has all but been discarded for two major reasons. First, if parents are accorded proxy consent to accept treatment, it could be argued that they may also refuse interventions for their children, even if those interventions are of established benefit or even life-saving in nature. Second, the primary obligation of the pediatrician must be to the child, and this stance may produce tension with the parent over the right to decide.[27] For both these reasons, recognizing proxy consent is now actively discouraged by the American Academy of Pediatrics.[28]

The Elements of Assent

According to Bartholome, assent in pediatric practice consists of four basic elements:

- Demonstrating respect for the child as a patient and as a developing person by assisting the child to develop an appropriate awareness of illness;
- Disclosing the nature of the proposed intervention and what the child is likely to experience, or truthtelling;
- Assessing the child's understanding of information and the factors influencing his or her evaluation;
- Demonstrating respect for emerging autonomy and the development of decision-making capacity by soliciting expressions of willingness on the part of the child to accept the intervention.[29]

This last point represents an obligation for care providers and may indeed be a stumbling block. The mere act of asking a child to accept an intervention forces the health care provider to respond to any dissent which is expressed. While most dissent can be handled with minor delays or apologies for the necessary procedure, asking the question may open a Pandora's Box from which it is difficult for the investigator to escape with patient rapport intact. If handled with appropriate sensitivity, however, the patient should emerge with an enhanced sense of mastery or control over the situation.

According to most ethicists as well as the National Commission for the Protection of Subjects of Biomedical and Behavioral Research, assent should be required for subjects at or above seven years of age.[30] At age seven, children are generally perceived to be capable of participating in their own health-care decision making. Assent or dissent should also be binding when used in the research setting but is always conditional upon parental permission.

In the practice of pediatric oncology, assent is not well studied. Oncologists' practices in obtaining assent from children are not well known. One published survey examined prevailing national practice on the issue of whether pediatric researchers should be required to obtain informed assent from minor subjects (with parental consent) as a precondition of the minor's participation in a research protocol; the results were widely variable.[31] At the heart of the issue rests the question of whether the proposed research is for therapeutic intent; if so, concerns about informed assent are less significant.

The other major difficulty with assent in pediatric oncology is that cancer center protocols may be too complex for true assent. One study of informed consent in the bone marrow transplant (BMT) setting revealed that neither parents and physicians felt that information was too complex but did find that a significant amount was lost to recall over ensuing days[32]. While parents did not relate information overkill as a side effect of the BMT protocols in the study, the generalizability of these results to pediatric clients giving assent is unclear and remains a target for future study. In the special case of Phase I trials, full informed consent requires discussion of all implications of treatment, including the possible benefit to future patients. Evidence clearly shows that children can understand and appreciate the importance of this information and thus should be included in the discussion.

Ethical Recruitment of Children into Research Trials

In the mid-1970's the National Commission (mentioned above) published specific guidelines concerning the use of children as research subjects. While concluding that research with children must obviously follow general ethical rules of research, the Commission enumerated the following special considerations.

First and foremost, there must be good reason to perform the proposed research with children, and the results of the research must be important to children's health. Second, careful attention must be paid to the determination of risk to the child. Third, the research must be governed by Institutional Review Boards (IRBs) whose objective is to determine the minimal threshold of safety, leaving the parents to decide the level of acceptable risk for participation. Fourth, parent/guardian permission and close involvement must be obtained. Fifth, assent/consent of the child must be sought at an appropriate age. On a case-by-case basis, children should be given the maximum level of decision-making autonomy permitted by their own capacity, and they must understand both the procedure and the concept of the invitation to help others voluntarily. Sixth and finally, the child's dissent must be respected unless the proposed research will provide the child with beneficial therapy that can't otherwise be obtained.[33]

The second point enumerated above deserves additional comment. The level of acceptable risk in research is determined by the potential level of benefit to be achieved by participation. For nonexistent or minimal risk, no prospect of benefit is needed. However, anything above minimal risk necessitates the prospect of some therapeutic potential. The ambiguity in this rule lies in the assessment of minimal risk, which is highly subjective.[34] The difficulty lies not only in identifying minimal risks but also in quantifying them; these decisions must clearly be made relative to each child's actual situation.[35] In practice, these issues are mostly encountered in the context of participation in Phase I clinical trials.

Ethical Justification for Children's Participation in Research

The basic ethical framework for research participation during childhood was embodied in the Ramsey-McCormick debate of the 1970's which culminated in the tenets developed by the National Commission. This seminal exchange is elegantly summarized by Bartholome and will not be repeated here.[36] For the purposes of this chapter, we will review key ethical points of the debate.

Participation of children in research involves a careful assessment of benefits and burdens. However, the scale is somewhat unbalanced, in that risk is only incurred by the participant while benefit may occur both to the child and to society. The best interests principle governs children's participation in research when the question is one of medical benefit to the child. Here the variability lies in the amount of potential benefit and risk, which is often subjectively quantified. In the case of nonmedical benefit to the child, socialization, communal values, and responsibility to become a moral being and citizen are called upon for justification for participation.[37]

Controversy arises when the discussion moves to situations of potential benefit for others. For cases of research without prospect of benefit for the subject, Ramsey lies squarely on the side against participation and cites respect for persons (unethical touching) as his justification. However, other theorists propose that the tenets of fairness and reciprocity can permit participation, as long as the risk won't impair the child's future development of capacities needed for individual self-determination. Essentially, this point is a conundrum because what is sought in research using pediatric subjects is knowledge about a class of persons whose character renders them incapable of giving or withholding consent. Therefore, some justification must be allowed for children's participation, or no information can possibly be gathered on this group of vulnerable people.[38]

Consent Forms

Any discussion of childhood participation in research must address the issue of consent forms. Multiple investigators have demonstrated that consent forms in general are too long and require an excessive education level to be clinically useful or even fair to patients and families. One particular study demonstrated that the average grade level necessary to understand a battery of different consent forms ranged from 11-14 depending upon the scale employed. The investigators discovered that concurrent verbal explanations aided family understanding, but that effectiveness could be maximally enhanced by scaling down readability to an eighth grade level.[39] Other factors mitigating the usefulness of consent forms are the milieu in which they are administered, and the time interval between diagnosis and form signing. Specifically, difficulty with readability and comprehension seems to be particularly high when the interval between diagnosis and consent/assent is short.

Psychological Factors Affecting Childhood Research Participation

Parents of children with cancer often have negative associations with enrolling their children in research trials and are hesitant to consent, at least initially. Reasons for this hesitation are as numerous as the individual families involved, but the most common perception seems to be that enrolling the child on a research protocol means that he or she will be "experimented on." These same parents are often unwilling to allow their children to choose to participate, often because of a fear of overloading their child with information and increasing anxiety at a time of maximal stress. Reluctance to participate in research is accentuated for minority patients, probably because of historical injustice to minority patients in medical practice and as research subjects. As a result of these factors, minority representation in research protocols is currently inadequate, meaning that results from any investigations have limited generalizability to minority populations.

On the other hand, there are a number of positive reasons to involve children in the decision to participate in research. Asking children for their assent for research participation gives them practice in making life decisions. It also increases their perceptions that they in fact do have some control over what happens to them and their bodies; imparting this sense of mastery is particularly important for seriously ill children, who often feel completely helpless to control any aspect of their lives. This sense of personal control that comes with choice can increase a child's commitment to the research project and thus improve his or her treatment outcome. Giving the child the choice also respects his/her individuality, autonomy and right to privacy. Finally, participation in research often results in increased self-esteem that comes with altruistic acts.

Many psychological factors have been identified in the literature which affect a child's ability to assent to research participation. Three principles of childhood development are clearly crucial: 1) as children develop socialization skills, they feel less pressure to acquiesce or conform to the wishes of adults; 2) as time perspective matures, children are able to stave off the need for immediate gratification; and 3) as children grow, their ability to manipulate concepts and understand ambiguity also grows.[40]

In addition to age-specific phases of development, other factors are clearly at work. These influences on the ability to assent to research participation can be understood to represent the child's social context, and include: relationship with the treating physician; intellectual capacity; previous decision-making experience; ability to consider consequences; impulsivity; and comfort with responsibility in deciding.[41] Obviously, none of these factors exists in isolation, and the specific interplay within each child and family unit will affect any particular child's ability or willingness to assent to research participation.

Ethical Objections to Securing Child's Assent for Research Participation

From an ethical standpoint, the primary objection to the process of informed consent/assent for the pediatric patient centers around the fear of information overload. Increased federal and legal pressures for excruciatingly detailed disclosure have resulted in longer and more complex consent forms and discussions, as mentioned earlier. Inundating patients and families with excessive information may trivialize the important issues, which become lost in the small details. To circumvent this potential problem, the information level should be determined by the investigator in a given clinical context; in practice, however, marked individual variation exists among pediatric oncologists as to the appropriate amount and content of information which should be dispensed.[42]

Pediatric End-of-Life Care

Over the last several decades, cure rates for pediatric cancer have improved dramatically due to advances in treatment and in supportive care. Because the prospects for a child diagnosed with a malignancy in 1998 are much more optimistic than was true even a few short years ago, most pediatric oncology patients and their families will not need to confront end-of-life issues. Nevertheless, almost one third of pediatric oncology patients still die. Palliative care for children is a science in its infancy, just as discussions of major ethical challenges at the end of life are only recently being extended to include pediatric patients. Gone is the paternalistic era of keeping children in the dark about dying, but providers are challenged to keep abreast of legal and ethical doctrine and, as always, to catch up with their patients and families in confronting these difficult issues.

Withholding/Withdrawing Life-Sustaining Treatment (LST)

At the point in a child's illness at which withholding or withdrawal of treatment becomes an issue, the ultimate goal of medical intervention is "to secure for the incurably ill child a death free of needless suffering".[43] The exact time at which the transition from providing to withdrawing life-sustaining treatment should occur is often hard to identify. And the difficulty is magnified in the case of a child with cancer, since previous emphasis has usually been on pulling out all the stops. In actual practice, physicians are often just as reluctant, if not more, to cross this boundary than are the child's parents.

Ethical and Legal Considerations in Treatment Withholding/Withdrawal

Though families and caregivers usually find it emotionally more difficult to discontinue treatment than to initiate it, no moral disctintion actually exists between the two entitites.

From an ethical standpoint, withdrawing and/or withholding treatment is permissible if the burdens of continued treatment outweigh the benefits or if the treatment is simply ineffective (i.e., futile). The benefits/burdens analysis is only valid as judged from the patient's perspective.[44] Decisions regarding withholding and withdrawing LST are generally made by considering a benefits/burdens analysis for a particular patient and removing any obligation to employ futile treatment.

Decision-making authority may be granted to the child, commensurate with his/her level of functional competence. Adolescent patients may actually execute "modified substituted judgment" in which they communicate their wishes to a proxy who then legally executes the decision.[45] In this situation, the role of family members in the decision-making process is inevitably diminished.

If prolonging the child's life entails a life dominated by suffering, the concerns of the family may play a larger role when decisions to withhold or withdraw treatment are made.[46] Research has repeatedly shown that parents who participate in decisions regarding withdrawal or withholding of LST routinely handle their child's death better and do not need to be protected from guilt in that situation.[47] However, the most prudent course of action is to consult an ethics committee when any decision to withhold or withdraw treatment is being contemplated.

The primary obligation of the health care provider must always be the child's best interest. When parents request withdrawal of LST, they are effectively withdrawing their consent for treatment.[48] Requests may at times be inappropriate, thus the health care team must ensure that parents possess accurate information about their child's disease and treatment before such decisions are honored. Conversely, parents and/or patients may wish to continue LST inappropriately, beyond a point of reasonable hope.[49] It is in this context that an understanding of futility becomes relevant.

Medically Futile Treatment

The definition of futility in the medical arena is a broad-based concept which is treated in detail elsewhere.[50,51,52] For the purposes of our discussion here, futility may be conceptualized as useless or worthless treatment which is incapable of improving any aspect of the child's life. Modern technology has created unrealistic expectations in families as well as in health care providers. Life can often be maintained for extraordinary periods, leading to misguided beliefs that underlying medical problems will be resolved if LST is initiated.[53]   Autonomy does not guarantee the right to choose useless procedures, but medical uncertainty can blur this distinction.

Futile treatment is not ethically justifiable, based on the principles of beneficence and justice (meaning misuse of diminishing resources).   Put another way, "interventions that are futile or offer extreme pain and suffering without a prospect of meaningful survival do not have to be provided, even if requested by the child."[54] If uncertainty exists as to whether a particular treatment is futile or not, shared decision making should be sought. The model of pediatric oncology practice may avoid some of these issues because of the early and long-term bonding that occurs with families in this specialty.

Unique Factors Affecting Withholding and Withdrawal for the Child with Cancer

In reference to withholding and withdrawing treatment, the culture of pediatric oncology produces several differences in decision-making practice and autonomy which merit consideration.[55]

First, children with cancer often have extensive medical experience. In addition to more first-hand experience with the medical system, these children may also have important specific knowledge to accompany their general maturity; both factors will contribute to their ability to advocate for themselves in critical situations. Second, the nature of modern cancer treatment itself dictates that the burden analysis needs to be measured in terms of psychosocial as well as physiological impact. A specific example of this concept would be to assign equal weight to time spent in the hospital as to specific debilitating physical effects. Third, children with cancer may exhibit unpredictable patterns of responses to treatment, ranging from better-than-expected with few side effects to the opposite extreme. Parental and/or physician biases may also threaten the child's well-being.

A final factor is that a distinction needs to be clearly drawn between the child who is incurably ill and one who is imminently dying. Some groups (i.e., specific religious factions and the AMA)[56] believe that LST should be foregone only if death is imminent. The trouble with this declaration is that actual pace and time of death are arbitrary and difficult to predict accurately. Instead of focusing on the nearness of death, the decision to forego LST should be based on whether the treatment is hindering the purpose or quality of life.

The Special Case of Nutrition and/or Hydration

No studies to date have been performed to assess the effects of dehydration on comfort in terminally ill children. Research in adults suggests that voluntary stoppage of eating and drinking occurs near death and reflects a natural bodily process. Rather than feeling hunger or thirst, dying people are generally more comfortable without intake, with fewer secretions and gastrointestinal symptoms.

Since controversy exists about the clinical effects of dehydration, especially in children, decisions again need to be made on a case-by-case basis. Perhaps the most sensible treatment of the issue is offered by Liben in an article on pediatric palliative care:

> ...it may be medically appropriate to withhold or withdraw hydration as a way of relieving specific symptoms (choking on excessive secretions, intractable diarrhea) in some terminally ill children. The critical question is not whether tube feeding is 'extraordinary' treatment but rather whether its benefits justify its burdens. Children, like adults, should have the right to freedom from the enforced prolongation of their dying.... The decision to impose medical hydration and nutrition should be made while considering the individual child's medical status, the parents' wishes, and the potential physical and psychological benefits and harms of therapy on the quality of life.[57]

Consensus Approach to LST in Pediatric Patients

Emotionally, the discontinuation of LST is often more difficult than non-initiation. In point of fact, not starting a treatment should be a more weighty decision, since the real issue is "not can we, but rather should we, embark or continue on a course of therapy which often has tremendous burdens with limited potential for success."[58] A practical solution is to offer a time-limited trial which is initiated after well-defined stopping criteria are agreed upon. This approach reflects the unpredictability of response to treatment without imposing undue burdens on dying children.

For situations in which children's best interests cannot be accurately determined, rational parents should be given decision-making authority. Children who have reached the age of assent and are capable of expressing a preference should be given choices and have their wishes respected. Physicians and other members of the health care team have no special authority to define the goals of treatment without imput from the child or parents. Put more elegantly, Leiken writes:

> ...if a minor has experienced an illness for some time, understands it and the benefits and burdens of its treatment, has the ability to reason about it, has previously been involved in decision making about it, and has a comprehension of death that recognizes its personal significance and finality, then that person, irrespective of age, is competent to consent to forgoing life-sustaining treatment.[59]

Palliative Care for Children

Palliative care involves comprehensive comfort care, inclusive of all interventions designed to relieve suffering, provided without curative intent. It involves any treatment measure used to control distressing symptoms and selected rationally in consultation with the child and parents to achieve well-defined objectives.[60] The approach combines multiple modalities to address the spiritual, social, psychological and physical needs of the child and family.

Despite the recent exponential increase in interest in the area of adult palliative care and hospice philosophy (as evidenced by the large proliferation of organizations providing hospice care in this country), a concomitant increase in pediatric palliative care and hospice services has not been witnessed. The fact that death is clearly less common in children than adults is not the only reason for this discrepancy. Families and health care providers alike exhibit tremendous variation in the state of readiness for transition to an exclusively palliative approach in the treatment of childhood diseases, even when the definition of palliative care is well-established and understood.[61]

Palliative care and hospice services for children enjoy universal appeal in the literature, yet many barriers exist to the actual provision of care. Some of these barriers include: 1) reluctance of parents and health-care providers to make a formal transition to non-cure-directed interventions; 2) lack of a broad knowledge base and practical expertise among pediatric caregivers regarding presentation of potentially fatal diseases of childhood, as well as differences in age, development and disease process; 3) lack of pediatric focus and training for community-based health professionals caring for children with potentially fatal illnesses; 4) dependence of children and their families on the tertiary care centers which have provided long-term care during chronic progressive illness, and the subsequent unwillingness of patients and families to transfer care to unfamiliar providers; 5) lack of experience among providers about pediatric pain and symptom management compounded with lack of formal assessment tools to assess children's needs in these areas; and 6) personal distress experienced by health care professionals due primarily to lack of support for and isolation felt by health-care providers who deal with dying children.[62]

All of these factors contribute to a greater or lesser extent depending upon individual circumstances. But perhaps the most commonly identified barrier is the notion that children are not supposed to die, and that referral to an end-of-life program signals failure on the part of the health care provider. As modern medicine has provided cures for many previously-incurable childhood illnesses and as technology has blurred the boundaries between life and death, the willingness on the part of providers to "give up" and transition to care from cure has diminished.[63] This is particularly true in the oncology field, where providers are often engaged in long-term relationships with families and may be unable or unwilling to step back and recognize when emphasis needs to switch away from definitive cure.[64]

In a recent international pilot study investigating mothers' experiences caring for their children with cancer during the palliative phase, researchers had trouble enrolling a sufficient number of families to complete the study even though the data was collected in institutions with more-than-sufficient numbers of terminally ill children. The study investigators postulated that the failure to identify children appropriate for palliative care stemmed from two basic areas: lack of open communication and ongoing discussion (both formal and informal) among members of the health care team about diagnosis, prognosis, treatment plan, and decisionmaking (i.e., the analogy of the horse in the living room); and disagreement about benefits versus burdens in terms of approaching families during times of maximum stress.[65]

This latter point essentially represents an ethical dichotomy between those who believe that parents of dying children are vulnerable and should be protected from any additional stress or loss of hope, and those who decry this approach as a paternalistic, disrespectful tack which deprives families of the ability to make their own decisions, give to others, or find purpose and meaning in their current experience.   The unfortunate end result of this discrepancy is that the majority of pediatric patients who could benefit from these services do not use them because they are not offered.   In point of fact, the mothers who were successfully identified and enrolled in the above study reported that open acknowledgment of their child's condition and prognosis gave them time to come to terms with the situtaion. Rather than robbing them of hope, they were given the opportunity to refocus the target of their hope from cure to the achievement of a pain-free state.[66]   One investigator sums up the situation this way: "The exclusion ... of patients and their families from receiving expert palliative care intervention and bereavement follow-up is an unjustifiable cause of profound suffering."[67]

Discussions and decisions surrounding end-of-life care need to include the family and the child in order to maximize adjustment to the dying process and comfort with the plan of care. In pediatric palliative care, only the individual child and family can determine what is good and right for them by calling upon their particular values and life experiences.[68]

Research with terminally ill children has shown that when information is presented in a developmentally-appropriate fashion, children are empowered if given decision- making authority over their own bodies and are often much more able to come to terms with their illness and death than are their adult counterparts. Possibly because emotional and psychological stress accelerates the maturation process, children as young as eighteen months who have cancer develop an understanding that death is irreversible; in contrast, this process begins after age nine in healthy children.[69,70] Indeed, some researchers challenge the notion that a child's conception of death is linked to stages of cognitive development at all. Instead, they report that in populations of terminally ill children, the conception of death seems to be related to experience with the illness and its treatment rather than to chronological age or cognitive stage.[71,72]

Furthermore, children must participate actively in the dying process in order to achieve mastery and control over their own dying. Providers must support these endeavors in order to help the child and family avoid helplessness, hopelessness and anxiety. Children have grief work to do and goodbyes to say, just as adults do. Shielding them from the opportunity to address these issues only robs them of autonomy and violates the concept of truthtelling in medicine.[73] However, when interventions directed at palliation are presented as a dichotomous option with interventions directed at cure, families and health care providers alike are asked to make a difficult, if not impossible, choice.

Do-Not-Resuscitate (DNR) Orders and CardioPulmonary Resuscitation (CPR)

One of the first steps in a successful transition toward palliative care for children is to step back from continuing aggressive life-saving attempts for critically ill children with poor prognoses. Just a few short years ago, finding DNR orders in children's charts was a vanishingly rare occurrence, despite consistent documentation that very few children are able to attain meaningful survival after sustaining CPR. Perhaps because the post-CPR survival rates for neurologically intact children are low but not zero,[74] DNR orders for kids are still found in the medical record far less frequently for children than for adults (33% vs up to 70% in one recent study).[75]

Most pediatric patients continue to die in the hospital, either in the ICU or in the operating room, and most are still receiving aggressive treatment up to the point of death. Age plays a role in that younger patients are less likely to have DNRs written, but this effect is difficult to assess separately from diagnosis, since causes of death are extremely different at different points in childhood.[76]

In the non-oncology population, DNR orders tend to be written late in the patient's course, such that most patients die relatively quickly after the orders are written, even though ventilatory support is not removed. Written orders usually follow assessments that further treatment is futile.[77]

In the pediatric oncology setting, DNR orders are somewhat more frequently obtained earlier in the clinical course. Though families may not be ready to hear the information or acquiesce to the concept until very late in the process, DNR orders are usually broached shortly after discussions of disease progression with or without experimental therapy. Patients who remain at home are often given letters signed by their primary oncologists to keep in their homes in the event that panic strikes at the end of life and families reflexively call an emergency squad. The letters explain to ambulance personnel that the child is not to be resuscitated; compliance with documents such as these has not been measured but appears to vary significantly.

Deciding to forgo CPR and accept DNR status is a major step for most families of dying children. Generally acceptance is a process occurring over a prolonged period of time and involving multiple discussions. Some ethicists argue that paternalism may rarely be justified in cases such as these in order to take the pressure to make a decision away from the family.[78] In practice, however, clinicians are extremely reluctant to circumvent parental authority in such crucial situations. Often the final go-ahead represents a turning point for the family at which denial is dropped and true acceptance of the child's death is achieved.

Terminal Sedation

With adequate provision of pallliative care measures, children should rarely suffer from intractable pain or other symptoms (such as dyspnea) at the time of death. Even with adequate education of providers and available medicines, though, an occasional patient develops a symptom which is refractory to standard palliative medical management. At that point a discussion of terminal sedation is sometimes undertaken.

Terminal sedation refers to an extreme form of symptom management which becomes the focus of care as obligations to assuage pain and suffering become more paramount.   When standard narcotic analgesia and all efforts to maintain consciousness while relieving pain have failed, terminal sedation has been used. Specifically, it entails a form of symptom control (usually intravenous infusions of barbiturates) designed to maintain an unconscious state until the moment of death.[79]

Used appropriately, terminal sedation is really only appropriate for a very small percentage of patients, and only after all other reasonable alternative methods of symptom control have been attempted. Applying the best interest standard here is tricky in children, as quality of life is difficult to assess, and severe, intractable symptomatology may color the child's ability to participate in decision making. Neverthless, terminally ill children need to maintain an appropriate role in the process because determining that a symptom is unbearable is, of course, entirely subjective.

Actually, the definition of refractory symptomatology is multifactorial; in addition to defining the physical symptom, the assessment must address the child's preferences for treatment, the child's capacity to tolerate the symptom, family/caregiver preferences and ability to tolerate distress, and a careful exploration of the person or people for whom the symptom is the most distressing. There are cases where it is "helpful to treat the child empirically for presumed distress, which...is essentially treating those who are witnessing the dying."[80]

The tone for the discussion of terminal sedation is set by the health care team. Family acceptance of palliative care in general and terminal sedation in particular is influenced by previous perceptions of poor medical care, poor communication with the health care team, and overall distrust of the people and the process involved.[81] By its very nature, terminal sedation has the risk of evoking fears that the child is being put to sleep, much as one would a pet. In order to facilitate acceptance of this form of symptom management, terminal sedation must be introduced along a continuum of palliative care options, not presented in isolation.   Additionally, families must never be put in a position to decide between comfort and keeping the child alive, nor must they perceive terminal sedation to be a response to external or societal pressures to end lives and/or limit medical expenses. Negative perceptions are more likely when discussions of this type occur in isolation rather than in process, or when the information is delivered by unfamiliar providers.

Physician-Assisted-Suicide (PAS) and Euthanasia in Kids With Cancer

The last step on the continuum from terminal diagnosis to death is to consider the prospect of hastening death in the terminally ill pediatric population. The difference between PAS and euthanasia lies in how the patient's life is actually ended. In PAS, the physician provides the method (such as a lethal prescription of barbiturate) but the patient takes the medication independently. In euthanasia, the doctor takes an active role by actually administering medicine by lethal injection or other method designed to kill the patient. A detailed review of this extremely complex and controversial subject will not be undertaken here, except to highlight the special features applicable to pediatric practice.

Most of the voluminous literature on this topic refers to adult patients, for whom statistics have shown that patients themselves and the public in general are more in favor of PAS and euthanasia than are doctors. In pediatrics, however, actual requests from parents to end a child's life are rare as parents usually find it quite difficult to let go. If such requests are made, undercurrents of anger and frustration can often be discovered and worked through.[82]

Arguments against PAS and euthanasia center around the fear of abuse of authority or outright coercion as well as the fact that focusing on hastening death distracts from attention to palliative care as a treatment option. These issues are even more salient for children, who are already more easily the victims of coercion and abuse of authority. Add to these reasons the difficulty of obtaining true informed consent (as we have discussed at length in this chapter), and the ethical issues become extraordinarily complex.

Just as with adults, one could argue that PAS and euthanasia might be ethically justifiable to prevent the "injury of continued existence."[83] The problem in pediatrics is that children can't voluntarily surrender their right not to be killed since they aren't yet competent. The hope of proponents of pediatric PAS/euthanasia is that any system put into place in this country will contain enough safeguards to prevent abuse of authority or death for convenience. But as the experience in the Netherlands has shown, numbers of patients who were successfully euthanized did not complete all the required steps of the screening process. Fears of the "slippery slope" in which expansion of authority will quickly lead to abuse of that level of authority is heightened when we discuss the potential that adult caregivers could be making decisions to put children to death.[84]

If PAS or euthanasia is ever to be codified for terminally ill children, efforts will need to concentrate on preserving the trust between the child, the family, and the doctor, since the primary function of the doctor is supposed to be that of healing. One could imagine that the availability of such techniques will forever alter the power balance between patients and physicians, and introduce a whole separate later of distrust. Other areas of focus will need to be on preventing abuse of the practice, preventing practitioners from becoming desensitized to killing, and continued adherence to hospice principles to discover medical, social, psychological and spiritual methods to address intractable pain and unbearable suffering.[85]

ETHICAL CHALLENGES IN THE CARE OF KIDS WITH CANCER

Having explored the basic principles of ethical decision making in pediatric oncology, we turn our attention in this section to areas of clinical care which are fraught with ethical challenges and subject to much debate in the current literature. These issues have the potential to compromise relationships between families and the health care team or, worse yet, detrimentally affect patient care. Though the following is by no means an exhaustive list, it represents concepts which should spark heightened attention for providers. Most of the problems discussed here can be softened or avoided altogether with thoughtful medical practice involving careful attention to verbal and body language and keen listening skills. Our intention is not to choose sides or to present an exhaustive overview of all areas of ethical debate. Instead, we attempt to reframe several key ethical issues in the context of pediatric oncology and offer some guidelines for respectful resolution of disagreement.

Paternalism

The modern medical paradigm has shifted from the era of "doctor knows best" to a time in which patient autonomy and advocacy are of prime importance. Nevertheless, children and families who come to tertiary care cancer centers seeking treatment for life-threatening illnesses are at high risk to become enveloped by paternalism because of the gravity of their situation and because they are, in effect, forced to trust unfamiliar "reassuring" providers.

Confidentiality and Privacy

The principles behind maintaining patient confidentiality in the pediatric oncology setting are no different than in any other areas of health care. However, most children with cancer are treated in teaching hospitals where large teams of people are caring for the patient. Many pairs of eyes fall on patient charts and cancer center protocol information. One solution to this problem is to limit information recorded on the patient chart, but this must be balanced with the need for the care team to have sufficient information to provide quality care.

For the most part, rules governing disclosure of patient information in the pediatric oncology setting are the same as in other medical circumstances: providers have a duty to warn potential victims under the principle of nonmaleficence, to maintain public health protection, to offer the benefits of medical attention to a third party, and to release information to sex partners but not parents (unless they're at risk).

Quality of Life Assessment

Very often in pediatric oncology, quality of life is used as a barometer when weighing the benefits and burdens of a particular treatment alternative or opting to continue or discontinue treatment. Adults can generally express their preferences about future states of life and health; when they are incapable of expressing those preferences, others can often estimate values and adaptation to future states by considering the history of the patient's preferences and lifestyle. In pediatrics, however, the life whose quality is being assessed exists almost entirely in the future, and expression of preferences is often not available.[86]

Research on the Dying Child

Despite the temptation to regard dying children as ideal candidates for novel research (especially for Phase I and Phase II trials), providers instead do well to remember that the dying child represents a subset of vulnerable children who, in fact, require greater protection from research abuses, not less.

Adolescent Patients

Legal and ethical debates about the appropriate age of consent for medical treatment or research participation are interesting and important, but both underestimate the complexity of the issues when it comes to caring for adolescent patients. In the first place, competence itself is not a static phenomenon; rather, it can be intermittent or fluctuating, and it may vary over time with changes in clinical condition.[87] Secondly, people are not static either: just as with adults, adolescent patients vary significantly in their ability to comprehend what is happening to them. Bioethical considerations are affected by individual cognitive decisionmaking abilitiy and by clinical stages of malignant disease. Care providers, therefore, need to be attentive to changing competence in adolescent patients, which may affect their conception of the good.[88]

Much biopsychosocial research has demonstrated that the age of consent should be lowered to fourteen years. However, blanket determination of age-related competence is less than straightforward because adolescent patients experience a number of confounding transitions which can have dramatic effects on their treatment choices. For one, patients are notoriously more concerned with their physical appearance during adolescence than during adulthood. While appropriate to the assessment of each adolescent's happiness and well-being, such preoccupations represent incompetence because they are not durable.[89] For another, late adolescents cross through stages of strongly oppositional behavior (often after the age of fourteen) and are capable of selecting treatment options as much for their ability to antagonize a parent as for achievement of a desired clinical effect. Finally, terminally ill or dying adolescents in particular often experience substantial guilt about failure to meet parents' expectations of health, and health care decisions based on that powerful emotion are often not in the best interests of the patient. These represent but a few of the many complex issues regarding adolescent patients; for a comprehensive review, the reader is referred to the 1997 Hastings Center Report.[90]

Disagreements Among Children, Families and Providers

Despite families' and health care providers' best intentions, mutual agreement about treatment or research participation is not always possible. In these situations, the obvious mandate is to protect the best interests of the child with cancer. Providers should first attempt to discern whether the disagreement stems from a breakdown in communication. Table 1 lists some common reasons for communication failure.[91] When analyzing these various factors, providers (and physicians in particular) need to be cognizant of the roles their own emotions and reactions may play in influencing professional preferences.[92]

Table 1: Causes of Communication Failure Between Parents and Providers

Parents are psychologically incapacitated at time of disclosure
Physician is detached or parent is overemotional
Communication does not occur at the parents' level
Parents receive misinformation from other sources
Parents and physicians possess inequivalent information

The next step in attempting to uncover the cause of disagreement is for providers to take a more detailed history. Often the source of the problem can be discovered by delving more deeply into family values, religious beliefs, cultural differences, and previous experiences with cancer or with the health care system. If conflict persists after these efforts, consultation with a hospital-based ethics committee may be sought to mediate the disagreement.

In the special case of an adolescent who disagrees with his/her parents, the primary allegiance of the health care team must continue to lie with the patient unless the adolescent's wishes are blatantly untenable or dangerous. Articulating the position of the American Academy of Pediatrics on caring for seriously ill children, Fleishman *et al* sum up this issue by writing:

> In the unlikely event that the views of the adolescent and parent cannot be reconciled through discussion and ethics consultation, we believe the physician should respect the adolescent's decision, informing the parents that the health care team cannot morally accept surrogate decision-making for a patient who is functionally autonomous.[93]

Alternative or Complementary Therapies

The decade of the 1990s has witnessed a dramatic explosion in the popularity of alternative or complementary medicine. Personal success stories abound, despite the lack of concrete evidence of efficacy in the literature. One major study revealed no difference in survival between patients receiving conventional therapy compared to those receiving "unorthodox" treatment; in fact, patients in the conventional group reported better quality of life.[94]

Patients with cancer are especially avid consumers of alternative medicines. A recent study of pediatric oncology patients in British Columbia revealed that 42% of kids used some form of nontraditional therapy and 24% of those did so without the treating physician's knowledge.[95] Numbers of this magnitude suggest that families will pursue alternative therapy with or without physican approval. Therefore, since the success of oncology treatment depends on enlisting parents and patients as members of the treatment team, the best approach is probably to encourage honesty about the use of such therapies. Unless clear evidence exists that the treatment is harmful, practitioners would be wise to avoid judgment.

If evidence exists that a given treatment has the potential to cause harm, the practitioner's responsibility is to protect the well-being of the child. Previous legal challenges have demonstrated that courts will side with physicians against parents for treatments known to be toxic, but judges won't pit physicians against one another in the determination of toxicity.[96]

Most products or services chosen by families raise very little controversy. Problems do occur with untested products whose potential toxicity is unknown and with products which require a physician's approval for procurement. Careful analysis of the benefit/burdens analysis is key here, and needs to include the risk of losing the parent trust if the request for compliance is refused. The most poignant down-side to these types of therapies is the risk of unfair capitalization on the grief and hope of desperate people. Parents facing the loss of a child to cancer are extremely vulnerable and willing to try almost anything to save their child's life. Many alternative treatments and practitioners are above-board and honest, while others are clearly out to take financial and emotional advantage of struggling families. It is hoped the the NIH-funded Office of Alternative Medicine will help to improve the science behind some of these treatments and weed out the others.

Refusal of treatment

When emotional scenarios of treatment refusal occur in the health care setting, it is hard for providers to remember that disagreement about treatment plans does not constitute parental abuse, neglect, or certain incompetence. In fact, conflicting judgments and decisions are inevitable in a model of shared decision making.[97] This is largely because estimates of benefits and burdens are rarely quantifiable and often subjective. Despite the best intentions of providers, the "element of subjectivity is ... irreducible. No advances in prognostic skills, physiology, or individual psychology can be expected to eliminate it."[98]   The following case demonstrates these ideas.

CASE REPORT 2

LS is a 15 year old Asian girl with high-risk T-cell leukemia, transferred from an outside institution for management of her disease. She had been well until two months prior to admission when she developed a Bell's palsy and huge cervical lymphadenopathy. Despite treatment with several courses of antibiotics and oral steroids, as well as an unrevealing lymph node biopsy, her adenopathy progressed. Finally she became acutely short of breath and was admitted to a local hospital after an emergent chest CT scan revealed a huge mediastinal mass with airway compression.

LS reports that she has lost about 15 pounds in the last 2 months, and has had intermittent fevers and night sweats. No one else at home is ill and there is no family history of leukemia or lymphoma. LS is one of four siblings from a rural town. She and her family came to the United States from Asia when she was a toddler; she has since been attending school regularly and speaks perfect English. Her parents, however, do not. She is a bright and articulate youngster who asks many good questions about her illness.

At the outside hospital, LS is diagnosed with T-cell ALL with CNS involvement. The diagnosis is explained to her and, through an interpreter, her parents. All demonstrate understanding of the diagnosis, the seriousness of LS's condition, and the need to start chemotherapy immediately. Because of her airway compression, LS receives her first doses of induction chemotherapy through a peripheral IV line. Despite appropriate prophylactic treatment, she develops severe tumor lysis syndrome and is transferred to the pediatric ICU for management of electrolyte abnormalities and renal failure. She undergoes dialysis, and after two days, is stable for transfer out of the ICU.

When it is time for her next dose of chemotherapy, LS and her parents adamantly refuse to allow her to have any more treatment. She has stopped taking the oral part of her regimen. She and her family state that they understand her diagnosis and the fact that she will die of her disease if she is not treated. They express, instead, the desire to seek herbal therapy to cure her. They mention several family friends who have been "cured" with herbs; none of these people has leukemia or is a child.

The hospital staff makes many attempts to reason with LS and her parents. An interpreter is brought in to reexplain all aspects of the treatment plan. Another Asian family with a teenager who has survived the same disease is contacted and agrees to talk with LS and her family. Several leukemia references and information booklets are translated into their language by volunteers. All of these efforts fall on deaf ears.

Finally, feeling they have no choice, the hospital contacts the county authorities. After failed negotiations with the appointed guardian ad litem and social worker, a petition is made to remove LS from her parents' custody. Despite being told repeatedly about the upcoming hearing, the parents do not appear at the appointed time in court and the judge grants custody to the county. On the same day, the patient's father travels to a nearby hospital and requests that his daughter be transferred. This request is granted.

At the new institution, LS and her parents are told that she will be receiving chemotherapy and that a central venous catheter will be placed for access. She and her parents agree to therapy. The following morning at the appointed time for surgical placement of the central line, however, LS refuses to go to the operating room. Numerous attempts to reason with her fail, and she insists repeatedly that the health care staff is committing child abuse by forcing her to take treatment against her will. She states that she understands that she will die if not treated but that it is her body and she accepts the risk.

The Relative Weight of Benefits and Burdens in Treatment Refusal

Most oncologic diseases are clearly fatal without treatment, so any decision to withhold is difficult to justify. Intervention by the courts is based on the principle that failure to obtain adequate medical care for a child is a violation of state child neglect statutes and is based on "standard methods of care."[99] Nonetheless, the right course of action is rarely straightforward. As we discussed earlier, the success of treatment in pediatric oncology depends on the development of an intimate working relationship between the family and the treatment team. Conflicts such as that encountered with SL and her family can jeopardize therapeutic relationships and exacerbate underlying problems.[100] Because treatment is ongoing over long periods of time and occurs primarily in the outpatient arena, a family can take the child and move away or the child herself can run away.

In addition to problems of client capture, decisions to pursue treatment may not be obvious because of perceived differences in levels of acceptable risk. Decision theorists state that difficult decisions require difficult decision rules. Indeed, the crucial issue may be to determine what constitutes acceptable cure rates for any given family to accept rigorous treatment. What may be an obvious choice in standard risk childhood leukemia with an average cure rate of 75% may not be so clear-cut if the child has a brain tumor with an expected five-year survival rate of 10%. Here again, the benefits/burdens ratio differs by case. When legal action is pursued, courts generally uphold parent rights to decide which risk is more acceptable, provided the child's life is not in immediate danger; for life-threatening illness, on the other hand, manslaughter convictions have historically always been sustained if treatment is not sought.[101]

Apart from the issue of survival, pediatric patients with oncologic diseases also face a number of handicaps such as amputation and effects of radiation therapy. Again, the relative weight of various outcomes is a personal choice and difficult to estimate from an outside perspective. During any given treatment, future interests should be more important than current experience, but children differ in their abilities to understand that current pain is the price to be paid for later benefit.[102]

Sources of Treatment Refusal

Unwillingness to pursue medical treatment may be expressed from several sources, namely the child/patient, the parent(s), or the health care team. Each places the treating physician in a slightly different ethical position, but all types are amenable to thoughtful conflict resolution in a supportive environment.

The Child: When treatment refusal is the choice of the child, the situation must be handled in a manner that maximizes the child's control over his body and/or dying process. If children are granted the right to assent to treatment, then dissent is a permissible response. If dissent occurs, the provider must assess the child's competence to make that type of decision. A finding of incompetence is usually easier to manage, albeit unpleasant at times. In the case of competent children who agree with their parents but disagree with the doctor, the general rule is that the doctor should acquiesce. When competent but in disagreement with parents, children's rights should be upheld and the physician should function as the child's advocate.[103]

Should children be asked to assent in cases of obvious survival benefit when providers have no intention of respecting refusal? Most opinions in the literature suggest not, except in the case of children with extremely advanced disease. These children require even more disclosure, since they'll likely discover the truth from other sources and be left with distrust of the health care team. Because of their experiences with disease and treatment, these children usually have an increased awareness of death and a better conception of individual benefits and burdens. Physicians treating terminally ill children who refuse treatment need to see themselves as advocates for patient self-determination.[104]

The Parent(s): Especially in cases where treatment benefits are likely to be small, parental refusal should not automatically trigger accusations of child abuse or neglect. Parents do not usually intend to harm their children. On the other hand, refusal of permission does not relieve the treating physician of duties and fiduciary obligations toward the child.[105] For the pediatric oncologist, the key decision is whether the benefit to the child is worth the emotional trauma of foster home placement during prolonged therapy. Such a disruptive course of action can be ethically justified only if treatment has a reasonable certainty of being curative or of inducing a long-term remission.[106] Historically, courts always side with a medical team requesting treatment, but will not pit one physician against another.

The treatment team: Reluctance on the part of the medical team to treat a child generally occurs in the context of withholding or withdrawing treatment, rather than a choice not to embark upon a treatment plan. Occasionally, however, staff feels that interventions are being done to, not for, the child. If a given intervention appears to resemble torture more closely than treatment, providers may refuse to participate in the treatment plan.[107] Open discussion is again of paramount importance, but reluctant team members should never be forced to deliver treatments they deem objectionable, even under the name of quality care.

Refusal of Treatment in the Research Setting

Situations do arise in which no approved treatment is available and a research drug offers potential benefit. If the child will die without this treatment, do the parents have the right to refuse? Yes, since informed consent for research includes a federally-mandated right to refuse, referred to as the "noncoercive disclaimer." Courts do not view this type of refusal as neglect.[108]

The Special Case of Blood Transfusions

The most common form of treatment refusal comes from Jehovah's Witnesses who refuse blood transfusions. Although a position based on religious grounds is not child abuse, the moral argument remains that of child neglect. Several special circumstances in pediatric oncology may again blur the lines: the child's prognosis may not be good; the treatment may be long, produce harmful side effects and result in chronic disabilities including second malignancies; and chronic life-threatening illness may result in serious psychosocial morbidity for the patient and family.[109]

Successful outcomes in these situations are best guaranteed by careful decisions to interfere with parental actions if and only if two basic conditions are met: first, that the actions will substantially harm the child; and second, that "the most likely result of interfering is that we will prevent the degree of substantial harm to the child that will occur without the intervention."[110] For the child with cancer, the usual goal of transfusion therapy is to permit the child to undergo further chemotherapy. Providers then need to determine whether this is, in fact, a beneficial outcome. Group statistics are meaningless in these situations – the outcome for each child is the main variable of interest. In some cases parents may actually be relieved if transfusions are ordered, thus preserving the therapeutic relationship and making the decision somewhat easier. In other cases, however, parents may consider their child to be damned; here, transfusion therapy undermines the supportive relationship with the child and family, and, more importantly, leaves the child to face treatment alone. Decisions capable of resulting in the latter outcome must give providers serious pause.

Conflict Resolution

The first step to restoring shared decision making is to clarify the goals of treatment with the parents and child. To reinstate a therapeutic context, the focus of this discussion should be shifted away from paternalistic application of universal decision making and toward decisions which are mutually agreeable. If framed correctly, parents walk away from these conversations with a sense of control and feel less need to act in an adversarial manner.

Conflict management is best done preventively, and providers need to realize that communication is not what is said but what is heard.[111] If, as our case illustrates, reasonable efforts at healing are undertaken but fail, numerous resources exist for more formal conflict resolution in the medical care setting. These include case-management conferences, psychology and psychiatry services, social work consultants, counseling, hospital-based ethics committee review, pastoral care, transfer of care to a willing provider (thus avoiding abandonment), and legal adjudication for refractory conflict. Providers who avail themselves of the particular resources in their own institutions can almost always avoid the legal venue.

CONCLUSION

The discipline of pediatric ethics as it applies to the pediatric oncology patient and family is a large area of interest and beginning exploration. In this overview, we have attempted to outline general principles of ethical influence on medical care for the child with cancer and the family. We have also chosen to focus attention on several key areas of ethical conflict or challenge, with the hopes of providing a background from which the interested reader can pursue further inquiry.

Despite the diversity of subject matter presented herein, several overriding themes are obvious. One is the extreme importance of soliciting the child's views and acting upon them whenever possible. Second, while general ethical principles can be applied to intellectual discussions surrounding care of the family, in actual practice most generalities do not apply and decisions need to be formulated on a case-by-case basis. Third, much research remains to be done to extend ethical inquiry into the pediatric realm, especially for some of the ethical challenges outlined here. Finally, whatever the question, the child's own perception of the issue at stake should occupy a place of foremost importance in the minds of pediatric caregivers.

REFERENCES

1. Fletcher JC, Dorn LD, Waldron P. Chapter 49: Ethical Considerations in Pediatric Oncology. In Pizzo, PA & Poplack, DG (eds). *Principles and Practice of Pediatric Oncology*: 3rd ed. Philadelphia/NY: Lippincott-Raven, 1997: 1284.

2. Buchanan AE, Brock DW. *Deciding for Others: The Ethics of Surrogate Decision Making.* New York: Cambridge University Press, 1989: 218.

3. Bartholome WG. Care of the dying child: the demands of ethics. *Second Opin* 1993; 18: 25-39.

4. Grodin MA, Glantz LH, eds. *Children as Research Subjects: Science, Ethics & Law.* New York: Oxford University Press, 1994: 29-30.

5. Sontag S. *Illness as Metaphor.* NY: Farrar, Strauss & Giroux, 1977.

6. Jonsen AR, Siegler M, Winslade WJ. *Clinical Ethics: A practical approach to ethical decisions in clinical medicine*, 2nd ed. NY: Macmillan Publishing Co., 1986: 176.

7. Grodin & Glantz, p. 86.

8. Buchanan & Brock, p. 219-228.

9. Buchanan & Brock,. p. 238.

10. Grodin & Glantz, p. 94.

11. Bartholome WG. A new understanding of consent in pediatric practice. *Pediatr Ann* 1989; 18: 262-265.

12. American Academy of Pediatrics Section Statement, Section on Hematology/Oncology. Guidelines for the Pediatric Cancer Center and Role of Such Centers in Diagnosis and Treatment. *Pediatrics* 1997; 99: 139-141.

13. Masera G, Spinetta JJ, Jankovic M, Ablin AR, Buchwall I, Van Dongen-Melman J, Eden T, Epelman C, Green DM, Kosmidis HV, Yoheved S, Martins AG, Mor W, Oppenheim D, Petrilli AS, Schuler D, Topf R, Wilbur JR, Chelser MA. Guidelines for a therapeutic alliance between families and staff: a report of the SIOP Working Committee on Psychosocial Issues in Pediatric Oncology. *Med and Pediatr Oncol* 1998; 30: 183-186.

14. Buchanan & Brock, p. 229.

15. Buchanan & Brock, p. 218.

16. Myers BA. The informing interview: enabling parents to 'hear' and cope with bad news. *Am J Dis Child* 1983; 137: 572-577.

17. Spinetta JJ & Maloney LJ. Death anxiety in the out-patient leukemic child. *Pediatrics* 1975; 56: 1034-1037.

18. Waechter EH. Children's awareness of fatal illness. *Am J of Nursing* 1971; 71: 1168-1172.

19 . Leiken S. A proposal concerning decisions to forgo life-sustaining treatment for young people. *J Peds* 1989; 115: 17-22.

20. Leiken, S. The role of adolescents in decisions concerning their cancer therapy. *Cancer* 1993; 71 suppl: 3342-3346.

21. Lesko LM, Dermatis H, Penman D, Holland JC. Patients', parents', and oncologists' perceptions of informed consent for bone marrow transplantation. *Med and Pediatr Oncol* 1989; 17: 181-187.

22. American Academy of Pediatrics Committee on Bioethics. Informed Consent, Parental Permission, and Assent in Pediatric Practice. *Pediatrics* 1995; 95: 314-317.

23. Beauchamp TL, Childress JF. Principles of Biomedical Ethics, 3rd edition. New York: Oxford University Press, 1989: 75.

24. Grodin & Glantz, p. 87, 94.

25. Brock DW. Children's competence for health care decisionmaking. In Kopelman, LM, Moskop, JC (eds). *Children and Health Care: Moral and Social Issues.* Boston: Kluwer Academic Publishers, 1989: 181-212.

26. Buchanan & Brock, p. 221.

27. Bartholome, 1989.

28. AAP, 1995.

29. Bartholome, 1993.

30. National Commission for Protection of Human Subjects of Biomedical and Behavioral Research. *Research Involving Children.* Washington, DC: US Government Printing Office, 1977.

31. Kapp MB. Children's assent for participation in pediatric research protocols: assessing national practice. *Clin Pediatr* 1983; 22: 275-278.

32. Lesko, 1989.

33. National Commission, 1977.

34. Grodin & Glantz, p. 51.

35. Freedman B, Fuks A, Weijer C. In loco parentis: minimal risk as an ethical threshold for research upon children. Hastings Center Report 1993: 13-19.

36. Bartholome WG. Ethical issues in pediatric research. In Vanderpool H (ed). *The Ethics of Research Involving Human Subjects.* Frederick, MD: University Publishing Group, 1996; chapter 14.

37. Grodin & Glantz, p. 86.

38. Grodin & Glantz, p. 91.

39. Grossman SA, Piantadose S, Covahey C. Are informed consent forms that describe clinical oncology research protocols readable by most patients and their families? *J Clin Oncol* 1994; 12: 2211-2215.

40. Koocher GP, DeMaso DR. Children's competence to consent to medical procedures. *Pediatrician* 1990; 17: 68.

41. King NPM, Cross AW. Children as decision makers: guidelines for pediatricians. *J Pediatr* 1989; 115: 10.

42. Kodish ED, Pentz RD, Noll RB, Ruccione K, Buckley J, Lange BJ. Informed consent in the Children's Cancer Group: results of preliminary research. *Cancer* 1998; 82: 2467-2481.

43. Freyer DR. Children with cancer: special considerations in the discontinuation of life-sustaining treatment. *Med and Practice Oncol* 1992; 20: 136-142.

44. Freyer, 1992.

45. Freyer, 1992.

46. American Academy of Pediatrics Committee on Bioethics. Treatment of critically ill newborns. *Pediatrics* 1983; 72: 565-566.

47. Clark FI. Intensive care treatment decisions: the roots of our confusion. *Pediatrics* 1994; 94: 98-101.

48. Clark, 1996.

49. Freyer, 1992.

50. Schneiderman LJ, Jecker NS, Jonsen AR. Medical futility: its meaning and ethical implications. *Ann Int Med* 1990; 112: 949-954.

51. Jecker NS, Schneiderman, LJ. Futility and rationing. *Am J Med* 1992; 92: 189-196.

52. Youngner SJ. Applying futility: saying no is not enough. *J Am Geriatrics Soc* 1994; 42: 887-889.

53. Ashwal S, Perkin RM, Orr R. When too much is not enough. *Pediatr Ann* 1992; 21: 311-317.

54. Leiken, 1989.

55. Freyer, 1992.

56. Council on Ethical and Judicial Affairs of the American Medical Association. *Current opinions: withholding or withdrawing life-prolonging treatment.* Chicago: American Medical Association, 1986.

57. Liben S. Pediatric palliative medicine: obstacles to overcome. *J Palliative Care* 1996; 12: 24-28.

58. Liben, 1996.

59. Leiken, 1993.

60. Cassileth BR, Lusk EJ, Guerry D, Blake AD, Walsh WP, Kascius L, Schultz DJ. Survival and quality of life among patients receiving unproven as compared with conventional cancer therapy. *NEJM* 1991; 324: 1180-1185.

61. Fernandez CV, Stutzer CA, MacWilliam L, Fryer C. Alternative and complementary therapy use in pediatric oncology patients in British Columbia: prevalence and reasons for use and nonuse. *J Clin Oncol* 1998; 16: 1279-1286.

62. Liben, 1996.

63. Liben, 1996..

64. Fletcher et al. 1997.

65. Davies B, Steele R. Challenges in identifying children for palliative care. *J Palliative Care* 1996; 12: 5-8.

66. Davies and Sttele, 1996.
67. Levetown M. Ethical aspects of pediatric palliative care. *J Palliative Care* 1996; 12: 35-39.

68. Liben, 1996.

69. Bluebond-Langner M. *The Private Worlds of Dying Children.* Princeton, NJ: Princeton University Press, 1978.

70. Nitschke R, Humphrey GB, Sexauer CL, Catron B, Wunder S, Jay S. Therapeutic choices made by patients with end-stage cancer. *J Pediatrics* 1982; 101: 471-476.

71. Batholome, 1993.

72. Susman EJ, Dorn LD, Fletcher JC. Reasoning about illness in ill and healthy children and adolescents: cognitive and emotional development aspects. *J Dev Behav Pediatr* 1987; 8: 266.

73. Bartholome, 1993.

74. Ashwal *et al.* 1992.

75. Lantos JD, Berger AC, Zucker AR. Do-not-resuscitate orders in a chlidren's hospital. *Crit Care Med* 1993; 21: 52-55.

76. Lantos *et al.* 1993.

77. Lantos *et al.* 1993.

78. Beauchamp & Childress, 1989.

79. Kenny NP, Frager G. Refractory symptoms and terminal sedation of children: ethical issues and practical management. *J Palliative Care* 1996; 12: 40-45.

80. Kenny and Frager, 1996.

81. Kenny and Frager, 1996.

82. Engelhardt HT. Ethical issues in aiding the death of young children. In Kohl, M (ed). *Beneficent Euthanasia*. Buffalo, NY: Prometheus Books, 1975: 180.

83. Faber-Langendoen K. Death by request: Assisted suicide and the oncologist. *Cancer* 1998; 82: 35-41.

84. Engelhardt, 1975

85. Faber-Langendoen, 1998

86. Jonsen, p. 187.

87. Buchanan & Brock, p. 217.

88. Leiken, 1993.

89. Buchanan & Brock, p. 222.

90. Weir RF, Peters C. Affirming the decisions adolescents make about life and death. Hastings Center Report 1997: 29-40.

91. Clark FI. Making sense of State v Messenger. *Pediatrics* 1996; 97: 579-583.

92. Aswal, Perkin, and Orr. 1992.

93. Fleischman AR, Nolan K, Dubler NN, Epstein MF, Gerben MA, Jellinek MS, Litt IF, Miles MS, Oppenheimer S, Shaw A, van Eys J, Vaughan VC. Caring for gravely ill children. *Pediatrics* 1994; 94: 433-439.

94. Cassileth, 1991.

95. MacWilliam & Fryer, 1998

96. Holder AR. Parents, courts, and refusal of treatment. *J Peds* 1983; 103: 515-521.

97. Bartholome, 1989.

98. Buchanan & Brock, p. 252.

99. Holder AR. Parents, courts, and refusal of treatment. *J Peds* 1983; 103: 515-521.

100. Ackerman TF. The limits of beneficence: Jehovah's witnesses & childhood cancer. The Hastings Center Report 1980; 13-18.

101. Holder, 1983.

102. Buchanan & Brock, 1989, p. 249.

103. Buchanan & Brock, 1989, p. 245.

104. Ackerman, 1980

105. Bartholome, 1989.

106. Ashwal et al. 1992.

107. Bartholome, 1993.

108. Bartholome, 1993.

109. Leiken 1993.

110. Ackerman, 1980.

111. Holder AR. Childhood malignancies and decision making. *Yale J Biol and Med* 1992; 65: 99-104.

10 DOES REIMBURSEMENT AFFECT PHYSICIAN DECISION MAKING?

Charles L. Bennett, M.D., Ph.D.
Tammy J. Stinson, M.S.

INTRODUCTION

Cancer care is expensive, with large expenditures being associated with new technologies and pharmaceuticals, supportive care modalities, and terminal care.[1] Almost one third of an individual's lifetime medical costs are incurred during the last several months of life. The high costs of cancer care raise important issues related to access to new cancer technologies. In particular, are all cancer patients equally likely to receive the expensive new medical developments? What is the relationship between patient's socioeconomic status and type of health insurance and the use of cancer therapies? Do financial arrangements between physicians and insurers affect the type and intensity of cancer care? Do these factors have an effect on the type, quality, and results of care in the clinical oncology setting?

Managed care has become the major form of health care delivery in the United States, with more than 60% of workers enrolled in Health Maintenance Organizations in 1998.[2] This trend is likely to continue to grow, either due to legislative changes or by economic forces. Until recently, oncologists maintained their fee-for-service status. But sweeping changes in Medicare reimbursements and the introduction of capitation have entered this field. Providing cancer care, which is inherently expensive due to the type of treatments, continuous technological changes, and high cost supportive care and monitoring required, presents a unique challenge to managed care organizations and the physicians that practice within them. The focus on cost containment is particularly difficult when treating an emotionally charged disease as debilitating and lethal as cancer. This chapter will consider the type of reimbursement strategies and changes in Medicare legislation that affect oncologists, summarize studies of the impact of cost containment on care, and discuss possible avenues to balance cost and quality of care.

MANAGED CARE PHYSICIAN REIMBURSEMENT STRATEGIES

How cost containment strategies affect the delivery of care has become a concern. Managed care organizations (MCOs) seek to limit expenditures, and one way they accomplish this is by designing reimbursement systems that reward physicians for practicing in a cost-conscious manner. This results in a shift in the financial responsibility from the insurer to the physician and their practice. In the general practice setting this typically involves incentives to limit access, either to specialists or to expensive tests and diagnostic procedures.[3] In the oncology setting, the trend appears to be heading towards capitation or case management mechanisms, allowing the oncologists to decide how to provide the best care for patients on a fixed budget.[4] Specific types of reimbursement strategies and how they influence care are outlined below.

Discounted Fee for Service

Under most managed care arrangements, specialists such as oncologists, are still reimbursed by "discounted fee for service" payments. The physician's work is defined based on episodes of care or specific procedures. The Medicare Resource Based Relative Value unit approach is one of the more sophisticated methods, accounting for the work effort and the overhead costs.[5] It is on this payment system that much of the inflation of medical care has been blamed. Under this system there is no restriction on the provision of services other than the ability to pay. It is assumed that this motivates physicians to provide more services in order to be able to bill for greater amounts.

Capitation Models

Capitation models are based on pre-paid coverage. A set amount of dollars are allocated per insurance member per month to treat cancer in a covered population. It is then the responsibility of the oncology practice to determine how to best care for the patients as whole within this budget. Oncologists assume responsibility for the costs of treatment and may also be responsible for laboratory tests and hospital services.[6] This type of system can be particularly difficult in the oncology setting, due to the wide variation in treatments, patient demographics and demand. It is possible to foresee that physicians may, at times, have pressure to restrain patients' access to services while being forced to work within a budget that is not adequate for their population's needs. Some efforts have been made to develop risk-adjusted systems, based on age and gender, but as of yet are primitive.[6]

Global capitation systems have been postulated to be a more successful means of managing costs while minimizing risk to individual physicians.   In this type of system a capitated budget is given to a large, multispecialty practice group spread over a geographic area. The advantage is that the risk is shared and less pressure is put on an individual physician when dealing with a particular illness or procedure. This also provides more resources for comprehensive care and education, which can lead to overall cost savings.

Physicians can limit their risk associated with capitation by obtaining reinsurance against losses or by including stop-loss provisions in their contracts.[6] Reinsurance protects the practice against patients that require exceptionally expensive treatment by covering charges in addition to the capitated amount. Stop-loss agreements are written into the capitated contract and limit physician liability per plan per year. The insurance plan is liable for any covered medical expenses in excess of the stop-loss amount.

Salaried Systems

MCOs have also investigated the use of salary systems as compensation for their providers.[5] In the private sector this has not been successful from the standpoint of cost-containment. Production has decreased and there is no incentive to monitor costs. There is also a decreased ability to respond to rapid change in the patient environment. Most salary systems now tie income to production and performance standards. Some have a partial salary system where income is negatively affected by excessive use of resources or failure to follow treatment guidelines.[3]

Medicare Reimbursement

With a high proportion of the patient population over 65, oncology practices are particularly vulnerable to the idiosyncrasies of the Medicare reimbursement policies. Medicare currently pays for chemotherapy drugs administered in the physicians' office based on the published Average Wholesale Price (AWP), although legislation has been introduced to decrease this amount to 95% of the AWP.[4]   This would be a detrimental change to physicians and the system. Acquisition costs do not cover the overhead costs of providing chemotherapy treatment, which can be partially recouped through full reimbursement of the AWP. Any overall savings realized under this change would be short-lived, as many patients would begin receiving chemotherapy as an inpatient as opposed to in the less expensive outpatient setting. Another limitation to oncologists of the drug benefit is that only drugs administered in the physicians office and intravenous drugs are covered.[4] Oral drugs, often preferred by the patients and less expensive overall, and self-administered drugs are not covered.

Impact of Reimbursement Strategies

A 1995 national survey revealed that over half of the physicians were associated with a managed care plan that put them at some level of financial risk based on the care they provide to their patients.[7] This leads one to consider the impact on patient care. Miller and Luft determined in 1994 that HMOs had lower hospital admission rates, shorter lengths of stay, similar rates of physician visits, and lower rates of utilization of expensive technologies than traditional fee-for-service plans.[8] Although the authors did not investigate whether financial incentive plans or other factors were involved in these findings. One of the most widely cited studies on this subject is the RAND Health Insurance Experiment, conducted from 1976-1981.[9] It found that annual expenditures in a group model HMO were 28% lower and hospitalization days 41% fewer than those in a fee-for-service plan. In same-physician studies, studies comparing utilization of services by patients with fee-for-service or HMO insurance treated by the same doctor, it was found that physicians used more services when treating patients for whom they will be reimbursed on fee-for-service basis than on a prepaid basis.[10,11,12] These services included diagnostic tests, hospitalizations and intensive care unit stays.

These studies were each conducted in the general practice setting, where "gate keeping" or control of specialist referrals is a ubiquitous component of managed care plans. General practice physicians have a great amount of latitude to affect costs in this role. But how physician reimbursement affects the oncology setting is a more difficult and subtle question.

COST CONTAINMENT IN THE ONCOLOGY SETTING

Evidence of significant variations in care for cancer patients as a function of financial considerations has rarely been investigated. Many policy makers feel that the life-threatening nature of the illness precludes the use of reimbursement as an important determinant of the magnitude of cancer care that is provided. Conversely, the widespread nature of financial ratcheting of medical care with respect to general medical care, newborn deliveries, and AIDS suggests that these policy makers may be misinformed. In this report, empirical studies which evaluate the relationship between reimbursement and cancer care are described.

Hematopoietic Colony Stimulating Factor Use

The hematopoeitic colony stimulating factors (CSFs), granulocyte colony stimulating factor (G-CSF) and granulocyte macrophage colony stimulating factor (GM-CSF) decrease the likeihood of neutropenic complications that result from chemotherapy, but their high cost lead to concern about their appropriate use. In 1994 and 1996 the American Society of Clinical Oncology (ASCO) published evidence-based, clinical practice guidelines for the use of CSFs.[13,14] In 1994, prior to publication of the initial CSF guidelines, and again in 1997, following the publication of the guidelines, ASCO surveyed its members regarding the patterns of use of CSFs and the degree to which preferences were consistent with recommendations published in the ASCO guidelines.[15,16]   In both time periods, a random sample of 1,500 United States physicians was evaluated.

The survey solicited data on respondents' patterns of growth factor use through hypothetical clinical scenarios. The survey also included questions on the impact of reimbursement considerations on use and choice of CSFs, existence of institutional guidelines on CSF use; and respondent sociodemographics, including specialty, and whether in a fee-for-service, HMO, or academic practice setting. The distribution of practice settings of the respondents was half being in fee-for-service settings, about one third in academic practices, and between 10% and 15% being in HMO practices. Less than one quarter of the respondents in both time periods worked with formal CSF guidelines or were in practice settings where guidelines were perceived to influence practice. Overall, the preference for CSF use was lower in 1997 ($p<0.05$). The most significant factor associated with stronger preferences for CSF use in both time periods was the type of practice setting. Compared to physicians in HMO or academic settings, physicians in the fee-for-service setting were significantly more likely to prefer CSFs ($p = 0.003$ for 1997 respondents and $p=0.001$ for 1994 respondents). Reimbursement considerations were less important in 1997. Only 20.9% of respondents indicated that choice of a particular CSF was dependent on prior experiences with denial of reimbursement (decreased from 27.8% in 1994, $p<0.005$), and 23.9% reported that their decisions about whether to use CSFs at all were influenced by anticipated denial of reimbursement (decreased from 34.7% in 1994, $p<0.005$).

Not surprisingly, when physicians face significant financial incentives to use expensive supportive care agents, their support of these agents is high. These studies raise concern over whether the rates of use of CSFs may be excessive in the fee-for-service setting, or, conversely, whether the rates may be too low in the managed care setting. While it is likely that dose intensity as well as schedule maintenance may be greater in the fee-for-service setting, it is not known if outcomes are better in the high intensity setting.

Measuring Financial and Clinical Outcomes in Oncology – the Prostate Cancer Instrument Panel Initiative

Performance measurement tools are integral to the provision of medical care today. The creation of health care "report cards" has been promoted by the desire to evaluate and compare provider performance for regulatory and purchasing purposes. The report cards, designed to identify factors associated with poor clinical outcomes, poor quality of care, or high costs, have been developed by managed care organizations, in large part for marketing, contracting, and profiling physician practice patterns, in which providers are rated on economic factors, such as fees and utilization. HMOs began to define sets of health performance measures in the late 1980s. The most prominent outgrowth of these efforts has been the Health Plan Employer Data and Information Set (HEDIS). HEDIS represented a pilot effort to develop a core set of reliable and valid health plan performance measures covering quality, access, patient satisfaction, membership, utilization, and finance. The aim is to track intra-plan performance and to permit appropriate inter-plan comparison.

There has been scientific controversy regarding the validity of report cards. There is concern that performance measures may not adequately adjust for differences in patients' severity of illness, when deriving severity-adjusted mortality or utilization rates, and certain hospitals may be unfairly penalized for treating disproportionate numbers of severely ill patients.[17] Health care is deriving new quality improvement methods based on business efforts.[18] Health care organizations have adopted business methods, using the terminology "instrument panel, " which provide frequent real-time feedback on the present status and future trends of selected patterns of care, utilization measures, outcomes, or patient satisfaction. A major aspect of this approach is that it provides essential, accurate, current information which can help improve medical practices. The panels are useful both to management, who frequently need to prepare responses to requests for information from insurance carriers, and to clinicians, who can improve their medical practices through more efficient use of resources. Instrument panels can be used to monitor the degree to which the clinical guidelines are adhered to, allowing for benefits in terms of both quality and efficiency of care.

An instrument panel approach was incorporated into the Citrus Valley Urologic Associated prostate cancer practice in Southern California, a group that is heavily capitated.[19] Predetermined prostate cancer guidelines for screening, diagnosis, treatment, and management have been developed and discussed with all of their referring primary care physicians. Real-time instrument panels measure outcomes, resource utilization, practice patterns, and patient satisfaction with monthly feedback given to each urologist in the group. The instrument panel- clinical guideline approach had several positive effects on the practice. Real-time feedback indicated that post-operative complications occurred at a higher than expected rate for three urologists. One chose to discontinue performing the procedure, and two decided to attend formal retraining programs. Consequently, as a group, bladder neck contractures decreased from 30% in 1993 to 4% in 1995, average length of stay for radical prostatectomies decreased by 1 day in the two year period, with average costs decreasing by 5%. Expensive practices such as autologous blood donation prior to surgery have been discontinued. The physician group as a whole has been supportive of this continuous quality improvement approach. Managed care organizations have viewed the program favorably and have negotiated additional capitated carve out programs.

The "report card" movement will undoubtedly affect the practice of oncology. Incorporation of clinical guideline efforts with "instrument panel" type feedback mechanisms can lead to improvements in patient outcomes, while providing more value for the health care dollar. Oncologists are likely to benefit from these efforts that stress improvements in care rather than hunting for "bad apples." While the driving force behind these improvement efforts appears to be an increasing reliance on capitated medical care, the end result may be lower costs, fewer episodes of treatment related toxicities, and improved physician performance.

The Relationship Between Out-of-Pocket Expenditures and Use of the VA Medical System for Prostate Cancer Patients

As overall survival in prostate cancer improves, more patients are developing advanced disease. The primary treatment for advanced prostate cancer involves the use of medical castration (LHRH analogs), agents that cost approximately $3,000 every three months. Fortunately for most patients, these costs are borne in full by most private insurance programs as well as Medicare. In some cases of advanced disease, additional therapy includes maximal androgen blockade with an oral non-steroidal agent is added. Despite the uncertainty over the potential benefit of these agents, the expense of $300 per month in additional pharmaceutical expenditures and the inconvenience of daily oral medications, physicians prescribe these medications to the majority of metastatic prostate cancer patients.[20,21] Medicare does not reimburse its $300 per month cost. Faced with out-of-pocket expenditures of $3,600 annually, most prostate cancer patients find it difficult to pay for the medication. Only in the Veterans Administration medical program is reimbursement for these agents included in the VA pharmaceutical benefit program.

Patients with prostate cancer were surveyed about their reasons for transferring their health care to the Veteran Affairs Health Care System (VA). While the VA is the largest integrated delivery system in the United States and serves the largest prostate cancer population in the US, the overwhelming majority of its patients are poor. We sought to evaluate whether the lack of coverage for oral anti-androgen therapy in the non-VA system might lead to transfers of care by low income Veterans with prostate cancer from Medicare covered providers to VA providers. While almost two thirds had private health insurance prior to their initial visit to the VA, only one quarter retained their private health insurance benefits after transferring care to the VA. The cost of oral anti-androgen therapy was the most common reason cited for transferring their health care to the VA, reported in over one third of the respondents. Other medical costs, such as co-payment for physician visits, ranked second (30.1%), a feeling that medical care would be better in the VA system ranked third (26.4%), and the co-payment costs of LHRH analogs ranked last (8.5%).

These findings suggest that many low-income Veterans with prostate cancer face financial barriers for medical care. While injectable LHRH agonists account for the largest pharmaceutical expenditure by the Medicare program, they are fully reimbursed and they therefore do not represent a financial barrier. In contrast, oral anti-androgens are not reimbursed by Medicare because their route of administration is oral rather than intravenous, subcutaneous, or intramsucular. Policy makers who are considering enactment of a comprehensive pharmaceutical benefit to the Medicare program will need to consider the resultant downstream effects on the VA and non-VA medical systems.

Financial Considerations and New Oncology Technologies: The Benefit of the Learning Curve Effect

High-dose chemotherapy with autologous bone marrow or peripheral blood stem cell transplantation has become the standard of care for many patients with relapsed NHL. The diffusion of this technology is unprecedented. Despite the rapid diffusion of this technology, there is comparably little reported information on the comprehensive costs.[22] At large programs, competitive financial pressures from insurers mandate that the costs of these procedures decrease over time, as newer centers compete with the established providers for patients. Most of this competition is based on case rate considerations, whereby insurers will refer patients to a center of excellence based on a preset negotiated payment per patient. To a lesser extent, the insurers force the regional centers to compete on quality and clinical outcomes, as well as costs. Nonetheless, it is likely that competition leads to pressures to decrease costs of care as well as improve clinical outcomes.

These considerations were evaluated at a single center, the University of Nebraska Medical Center.[23,24] This center is one of the largest referral centers for lymphoma in the United States. It was found that the costs of care for Non-Hodgkin's lymphoma patients who received an autologous stem cell transplant decreased by 25% between 1987 and 1991, while the average inpatient stay decreased from 45 days to 38 days. During this evaluation period, the use of hematopoietic colony stimulating factors was a major reason for shortened periods of neutropenia, earlier discharge, and significant cost savings. In contrast, with increased economic pressures in 1991, the duration of the transplant admission decreased further to 11.9 days by 1995. In addition, the comprehensive costs of care decreased 14% by 1991, and an additional 51% between 1991 and 1995 for patients with Non-Hodgkin's lymphoma. The major determinant of lower costs was the 80% decrease in transplant hospitalization room costs. As a result of dramatic decreases in dollars spent on all inpatient transplant resources, and the relatively stagnant costs associated with outpatient and additional inpatient resources over time, outpatient costs increased relative to the decreasing transplant hospitalization costs. Total outpatient costs made a somewhat disproportionate contribution of only 14% of the total experience in 1989, 26% by 1992, but 49% by 1995.

Lower health care costs over time have been attributed to three potential factors: 1) hospitals that have treated large numbers of patients are further along on the learning curve in caring; 2) a referral system has been established so that as hospitals gain experience, they admit patients who are better candidates for the procedure; or 3) technologic improvements have occurred.[25]

The results have important policy implications with respect to the debate over regionalization of care. Technologic advances can be efficiently disseminated through educational programs, scientific meeting presentations, and journal publications and would not require regionalization of services in most cases. Conversely, effects that are associated with organizational changes require large amounts of capital expenditures for procurement of facilities and experienced personnel. Geographic areas with large numbers of transplant centers are unlikely to fully realize these organizational benefits at each of the centers and regionalization is likely to be an efficient alternative. The striking decrease in costs since 1991 reported from the University of Nebraska suggests that policy makers would be wise to limit the diffusion of transplant programs to large centers of excellence.

Financial Considerations and Oncology: The Potential Downside of Rapid Adoption of a New Technology

While stem cell transplant program administrators almost always negotiate case rates for patients undergoing these procedures, as described above, these competitive financial pressures can potentially lead to worsening of clinical outcomes, despite significant cost savings. Such an example potentially exists in the case of allogeneic stem cell transplantation for hematologic malignancies. The first allogenic peripheral blood stem cell transplants were performed in the early 1990s, and as of April 1997, it is estimated that 2,500 allogeneic peripheral blood stem cell transplantations have been performed worldwide. However, only three large transplant centers have performed over 100 allogeneic peripheral blood stem cell transplant procedures with most of the other centers having performed less than 50.

Early assessments of value of stem cell transplantation pose unique methodologic problems.[26] First, dissemination of new technologies is generally preceded by assessments of efficacy in the ideal setting, while effectiveness estimates in the usual practice setting occur at a later period of time. Second, while short-term costs can be estimated in clinical trials, long-term costs are unknown. Despite these limitations, "the assessment of value early in the development of new clinical strategies should be a prerequisite to their dissemination."[26]

Dramatic improvements in hematopoietic recovery times, as noted in several phase II clinical trials, led to the rapid dissemination of autologous peripheral blood stem cell transplantation over autologous bone marrow transplantation.[27] An additional consideration was the expectation of lower costs for the autologous peripheral blood stem cell transplant procedure. Similar clinical and economic considerations may apply to allogeneic stem cell transplantation.

Concerns exist about the comparative clinical and economic benefits compared to allogeneic bone marrow transplantation. At the University of Nebraska program, patients who undergo an allogeneic peripheral blood stem cell transplantation for hematologic malignancies have 5.5 fewer days until neutrophil recovery, 11 fewer days until platelet recovery, and 5 days shorter hospitalizations than for similar patients who undergo an allogeneic bone marrow transplantation.[28] In addition, these individuals achieve a 19% short-term cost savings as measured from the time of stem cell harvest until 100 days following the stem cell transplantation. A second study from France also found that among 51 patients enrolled in a randomized phase III clinical trial, the duration of severe neutropenia was shortened by 5 days, severe thrombocytopenia by 10 days, and costs were reduced by 20% with alloPBSCT.[29] However, clinicians remain concerned that long-term costs and clinical outcomes, as measured from day 100 onward, may be poorer for individuals who undergo an allogeneic peripheral blood stem cell transplant, primarily because of concern that chronic graft versus host disease may be worse for these individuals.

These results have direct policy implications. For autologous stem cell transplantation, evidence of clinical benefits and cost savings in phase II trials resulted in rapid acceptance of autologous peripheral blood stem cell transplantation, necessitating early closure of an important phase III randomized trial which included clinical and economic comparisons of the two procedures. If the usual scientific process of evaluating new technologies by phase II and subsequent phase III trials is not followed, knowledge of the long term results of the two types of allogeneic stem cell transplantation could be jeopardized. If the switch to peripheral blood stem cell transplant occurs based on short term economic results, more chronic GVHD and higher long term costs could result. Also, more toxic conditioning regimens, that might improve the cure rate, would be penalized due to longer initial hospitalizations and higher short term costs.

Medicare Reimbursemant Policies: The effect on the Use of Oral Chemotherapy Agents

Currently used options for salvage therapy for epithelial ovarian cancer include intravenously administered paclitaxel or topotecan and orally administered altretamine or etoposide. The response rates for these agents are similar (14-26%) while the type and incidence of adverse events differs. Under current legislation, Medicare will reimburse intravenous outpatient chemotherapy regimens only or oral regimens with a marketed intravenous formulation, despite that 89% of cancer patients prefer oral therapies. To compare the out of pocket costs and costs to the Medicare system, a cost minimization analysis of treatment with these agents was conducted utilizing published phase II and phase III data.[30] The total cost of treatment was $15,767 for paclitaxel, $18,635 for topotecan, $4,477 for altretamine, and $5,016 for etoposide.   The out of pocket costs to the patient were $83, $37, $4,477 and $6, respectively.

The impact of Medicare reimbursement policies has also been noted in other areas of cancer care. Oral antiemetics are only reimbursed under very specific and limited circumstances. Only one dose is covered with pre-chemotherapy treatment with Medicare-approved oral antineoplastics, when necessary to ensure oral absorption. Oral antiemetics given with intravenous chemotherapy agents in the outpatient setting are not covered.[31]

While a physician's first consideration in choosing a therapy for their patients is efficacy and toxicity, current Medicare reimbursement policies restrict patient options for cancer care. As Medicare adopts managed care and HMOs into the management of patient care, cost-effectiveness will likely become an important consideration in the treatment of cancer. Because long-term survival of ovarian cancer patients following salvage therapy is extremely poor, it is important to consider factors affecting quality of life, such as the convenience of therapy administration, the incidence of discomfort and debilitating adverse events, and stress caused by significant out of pocket costs. While there is evidence of patient preferences for oral versus intravenous administration of chemotherapeutic agents, our cost models suggest that when efficacy and toxicity are equal, the more expensive intravenous agents may be used over less expensive oral alternatives because of concern over out-of-pocket costs to the patient. Although the influx of managed care in Medicare may provide more options and greater cost savings, less than half of the current Medicare patients are enrolled in these programs.

CONCLUSION

The economics of medicine directly influence the practice of physicians and, overall, of oncology today. In this paper, empirical findings indicate that competitive economic pressures can lead to dramatic improvements in clinical outcomes, premature adoption of new technologies with the potential for poorer clinical outcomes, and transfers of medical care between different health care sectors. It is therefore impossible to make a blanket statement that competitive financial pressures are likely to lead to poorer medical care, or even improved better care. Each clinical and economic medical situation represents a unique set of circumstances. Nonetheless, policy makers would be wise to acknowledge the direct relationship between financial considerations and clinical care in oncology.

REFERENCES

1. Smith TJ. Role of granulocyte and granulocyte macrophage colony stimulating factors in clinical practice: Balancing clinical and economic concerns. American Society of Clinical Oncology Educational Book. 35th Annual Meeting. 1999: 275- 299.

2. McIntosh H. Managed care brings major changes to cancer care. J Natl Cancer Inst 1995; 87:784-86.

3. Hellinger FJ. The impact of financial incentives on physician behavior in managed care plans: A review of the evidence. Med Care Res Review 1996; 53(3):294-314.

4. Bailes JS. Health care economics of cancer in the elderly. Cancer 1997; 80:1348-50.

5. Ogrod ES. Compensation and quality: A physician's view. Health Affairs 1997; 16(3):82-86.

6. Simon CJ and Emmons DW. Physician earnings at risk: An examination of capitated contracts. Health Affairs 1997; 16(3):120-26.

7. Health News Daily. 1995. Half of US physicians are associated with risk insurance plans, Nov 13, p. 4.

8. Miller R, Luft HS. Managed care plan performance since 1980. J Am Med Assoc 1994; 271:1512-19.

9. Manning WF, Leibowitz A, Goldberg FA, Rogers WH, Rogers JP. A controlled trial of the effects of a prepaid group practice on use of services. N Eng J Med 1984; 310:1505-10.

10. Clancy CM, Hillner BE. Physicians as gatekeepers: The impact of financial incentives. Arch Int Med 1989; 149:917-20.

11. Greenfield S, Nelson EC, Zubkoff M, et al.   Variations in resource utilization among medical specialties and systems of care. J Am Med Assoc 1992; 267:1624-30.

12. Rappaport J, Gehlback S, Lemeshow S, Teres D. Resource utilization among intensive care patients: Managed care versus traditional insurance. Arch Int Med 1992; 152:2207-12. .

13. American Society of Clinical Oncology. American Society of Clinical Oncology recommendations for the use of hematopoietic colony stimulating factors: Evidence based clinical practice guidelines. J Clin Onc 1994; 12: 2471- 2508.

14. Update of recommendations for the use of hematopoietic colony stimulating factors: Evidence-based clinical practice guidelines. J Clin On 1996; 14: 1957- 1960.

15. Bennett CL, Smith TJ, Weeks JC et al. Use of hematopoietic colony stimulating factors: The American Society of Clinical Oncology Survey. J Clin Onc 1997; 14: 2511- 2520.

16. Bennett CL, Somerfield M, Feinglass J, Smith TJ. Decrease in misuse/overuse of hematopoietic colony stimulating factors for solid tumors and lymphomas: Results from ASCO Surveys Related to the 1994 and 1996 ASCO CSF Guidelines. Proceedings of ASCO 1998; 17: 421a.

17. Park RE, Brook RH, Kosecoff J et al. Explaining variations in hospital death rates. Randomness, severity of illness, quality of care. JAMA 1990; 264: 484- 490.

18. Bataladan P, Nelson E, Roberts J. Linking outcomes measurement to continual improvement: the serial "V" way of thinking about improving clinical care. Jt Comm J Qual Improv 1994; 20: 167- 80.

19. Ullman M, Metzger CK, Kuzel T, Bennett CL. Performance measurement in prostate cancer: Beyond report cards. Urology 1996; 47: 356- 65.

20. Bennett CL, Tosteson TD, Schmitt B, Weinberg PD, Ernstoff MS, Ross SD. Maximum androgen blockade with medical or surgical castration in advanced cancer: A meta-anlysis of nine published randomized controlled trials and 4128 patients using flutamide. Prostate Cancer and Prostatic Diseases 1999; 2: 4-8.

21. Eisenberger MA, Blumenstein BA, Crawford ED et al. Bilateral orchiectomy with or without flutamide for metastatic prostate cancer. NEJM 1998; 339: 1036-42.

22. Waters TM, Bennett CL, Pajeau TS, Sobocinski KA, Klein JP, Rowlings PA, Horowitz M. The Costs and Cost-Effectiveness of Bone Marrow and Peripheral Blood Stem Cell Transplantation: What Do We Know? Bone Marrow Transplant 1998; 21:641-50.

23. Bennett CL, Armitage JL, Armitage GO, et al. Costs of care and outcomes for high-dose therapy and autologous transplantation for lymphoid malignancies: Results from the University of Nebraska 1987-1991. J Clin Oncol 1995; 13:969-973.

24. Freeman MB, Vose JM, Bennett CL et al. Costs of Care for High-Dose Therapy and Autologous Transplantation for Non-Hodgkin's Lymphoma: Results From the University of Nebraska Medical Center 1989 Through 1995; Bone Marrow Transplantation 1999; in press.

25. Luft HS, Bunker JP, Enthoven AC. Should operations be regionalized? The empirical relation between surgical volume and mortality. N Engl J Med 1979; 301:1364-1369.

26. Welch HG. Valuing clinical strategies early in their development. Annals of Int Med116: 263-4; 1992.

27. Pavletic ZS, Bishop MR, Tarantolo SR, et al. Hematopoietic recovery after allogeneic blood stem cell transplantation compared to bone marrow transplantation in patients with hematologic malignancies. J Clin Oncol 1997; 15:1608-13.

28. Bennett CL, Waters TM, Stinson TJ et al. Valuing Clinical Strategies Early in Development: A Cost Analysis of Allogeneic Peripheral Blood Stem Cell Transplantation.   Bone Marrow Transplantation 1999; in press.

29. Blaise D, Kuentz M, Fortanier C, et al. Randomized trial of lenograstim-primved blood cell versus bone marrow allogeneic transplantation: Comparison of haematological recovery and socioeconomic evaluation. Proceedings of the American Society of Hematology 1998; 557a.

30. Bennett CL, Stinson TJ, Yang T, Lurain JR.   The Effect of Reimbursement Policies on the Management of Medicare Patients with Refractory Ovarian Cancer. Sem Oncol 1999; 26(1) Suppl A:34-39.

31. Ignoffo RJ.   Medicare Reimbursement for Oral Antiemetics in Management of Chemotherapy-Induced Emesis. Am J Health-Syst Pharm 1997; 54:830-31.

Index